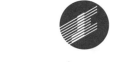

Joint Commission

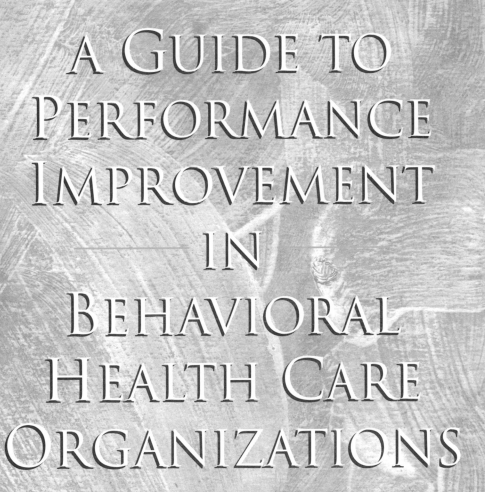

A Guide to Performance Improvement in Behavioral Health Care Organizations

Joint Commission Mission
The mission of the Joint Commission on Accreditation of Healthcare Organizations is to improve the quality of care provided to the public through the provision of health care accreditation and related services that support performance improvement.

Joint Commission educational programs and publications support, but are separate from, the accreditation activities of the Joint Commission. Attendees at Joint Commission educational programs and purchasers of Joint Commission publications receive no special consideration or treatment in, or confidential information about, the accreditation process.

Dedication

This book is dedicated to Linda Striggles, a Joint Commission surveyor who died March 24, 1995, on her way home from a survey. Linda was a source of motivation, pride, and inspiration to all who knew her. Using her intelligence, humor, and an obsession for detail, she was tireless in helping behavioral health care organizations improve the quality of care and services provided to their clients. It seems most fitting to those of us who knew and worked with her to dedicate this book on performance improvement to her.

Contents

Introduction

Driven by its mission "to improve the quality of care provided to the public through the provision of health care accreditation and related services that support performance improvement," the Joint Commission has incorporated contemporary knowledge about organization excellence into its quality improvement approach or framework. This framework is designed to help health care organizations achieve high-quality care, optimal outcomes, and efficient use of resources.

Providing high quality care is challenging—it means that treatment is efficacious and appropriate, available when needed, and delivered in a timely fashion. Equally important, it is provided in a respectful and caring manner. It is also effective, safe, efficient, and well coordinated over time and across practitioners and settings.

Behavioral health care* organizations that systematically improve the quality of care delivery can expect superior care outcomes, more competitive costs, and high levels of client satisfaction. Delivery of high-quality care is

---

* Henceforth, when the term *behavioral health care* is used, it includes mental health, chemical dependency, forensic, and mental retardation/developmental disabilities services unless otherwise noted.

directly related to performance of critical organization systems, and the effective, coordinated performance of multiple jobs and tasks.

In developing this quality improvement framework, the Joint Commission has carefully synthesized a wide range of available theories, methods, and tools, and added its own experience. This approach gives professionals methods to systematically and scientifically enhance care processes and their outcomes. The framework has grown out of the long-standing search for quality and the efforts of literally hundreds of health care organizations and professionals.

The framework emphasizes total quality management and continuous quality improvement strategies. These strategies stress the importance of leadership, and understanding external and internal customer needs. They also include opportunities for outcomes-driven design of new products and services, broad use of measurement systems, data-driven performance assessment, and systematic design and redesign of important organization processes and functions.

The framework's primary goals are

- to emphasize the link between an organization's performance of important functions and its care outcomes, the costs to achieve these outcomes, and judgments about the quality and value of its services;
- to illustrate how an organization can mesh the rich variety of concepts, methods, and strategies developed independently over the past several decades into an operational performance improvement system relevant to health care; and
- to demonstrate that the effectiveness with which an organization manages its relationship with the external environment is as important to the fulfillment of its mission as the effectiveness with which it manages its internal environment.

This book describes the framework's application to behavioral health care organizations. Initially, it provides an overview of the principles and history on which the framework is built, and introduces the primary components of the framework, which include

- the external environment, including the political, social, economic, and other forces in society that influence how a mental health, chemical dependency, forensic, mental retardation/ developmental disabilities organization delivers service and fulfills its mission;
- the internal environment, particularly the governance, management, clinical, and support activities that affect care delivery and outcomes; and
- the cycle for improving performance—a practical method for improving processes.

Subsequent chapters explore each stage of the improvement cycle and present examples adapted from a variety of services and settings.

This book is a practical and pragmatic guide. It can be used to acquire an overview of performance improvement concepts and methods. It can also be used as a resource for organizations to help carry out their improvement activities.

▣ Summary

This improvement framework presents many challenges to health care organizations, particularly in behavioral health care, including becoming more individual-focused, redesigning care processes, promoting collaborative teamwork, systematically measuring and assessing performance, and encouraging risk taking and experimentation. The ability to proactively and effectively manage quality is perhaps the only way that organizations will prosper in the face of stringent resource constraints and increasing demands for better care and service outcomes.

1

Overview

"The long-range contribution of statistics depends not so much upon getting a lot of highly trained statisticians into industry as it does on creating a statistically minded generation . . . who will in any way have a hand in developing and directing processes of tomorrow."

—*Statistical Method from the Viewpoint of Quality Control*

- Introduction
- Underlying Principles
- Components of the Framework for Improving Performance
- Chapter Summary

▣ Introduction

There are extraordinary forces at work reshaping health care today in the United States. Everywhere we look—newspapers, television news broadcasts, magazines, health care publications—commentaries highlight the intense concern about the future of health care. Key issues include the availability, quality, and value of health care. These concerns are shared by the recipients of care, care providers, the public, purchasers, payers, accreditors, regulators, and others. These concerns are fueling unprecedented efforts to understand and improve how health care is delivered.

In the past decade, cost-containment strategies, including prospective payment plans, capitation, and managed care, have dramatically reshaped the delivery of health care services. Managed care has grown from modest beginnings to become the dominant form of care of medically insured people in the United States. The emerging trends in health care delivery have included

- movement from hospital-based toward community-based care;
- expansion of gatekeeping functions and case management services for cost containment and to further integrate care; and
- design of shared risk and collaborative reimbursement models.

More recent developments have also included a strong movement toward outcomes research and disease management concepts.

It is in this context that behavioral health services stand, facing increasing scrutiny and oversight. Behavioral health care* organizations may have been particularly vulnerable to service "carve outs," cost containment, and decreasing accessibility, in part, because their work involves a gray zone of "softer" science (that is, human behavior and the management of thoughts and feelings). It is important to note that there has been little empirical research or objective data demonstrating both the effectiveness and efficiency of behavioral health services, and much of what does exist has not been systematically applied in clinical areas. Performance data is vital now, when decision makers and policy makers, payers, and the individuals served and their families are demanding that organizations provide information to demonstrate the value of their services by measuring their outcomes. Behavioral health care is also seeking an equal position in reimbursement under national health care reform.

Therefore, the missions of the Joint Commission and the behavioral health organization seeking accreditation are strongly aligned. Both are driven

---

* Henceforth, when the term *behavioral health care* is used, it includes mental health, chemical dependency, forensic, and mental retardation/developmental disabilities services unless otherwise noted.

to improve the quality of care provided to the public. Since the inception of its mental health accreditation program in the 1970s (developmentally disabled programs in 1971, psychiatric facilities in 1972, substance abuse programs in 1974, and community mental health centers [CMHCs] in 1976), the Joint Commission has carried out this mission through several ongoing activities:

- Developing standards and gaining national consensus on standards for mental health, chemical dependency, and developmental disabilities;
- Evaluating organizations to determine compliance with the standards;
- Educating and leading efforts in performance improvement and other issues central to quality; and
- Developing process and outcome indicators useful to organizations and the Joint Commission in evaluating the level of performance of important functions.

▣ Underlying Principles

One product of the Joint Commission's activities is a framework for improving performance. This framework rests on several related, interlocking principles. These principles focus on the purpose of health care, how health care is delivered, and how health care is improved. These principles are briefly reviewed here. In the remaining chapters of this book, these principles will be demonstrated in case studies and discussion.

The Purpose of Health Care

The central purpose of health care is to maximize the health and comfort of the people served and provide the highest quality care in a cost-effective manner, regardless of the specific setting or service. Many variables (from both the external and internal environments) influence the success of an organization in achieving this central purpose. For example, competence of the clinicians who provide care, the availability of adequate staffing, and the individual's or family's ability to participate in the client's care all affect outcomes.

Behavioral health care organizations also face a unique challenge. Behavioral health care outcomes are difficult to develop and assess, perhaps by virtue of their broad treatment perspective and the extent to which care is influenced by social, environmental, and medical factors. The work of behavioral health care organizations also spans a huge array of services (for example, mental health, chemical dependency, mental retardation/developmental disabilities, and post-acute acquired brain injury services) and care settings (for example, inpatient, residential, supervised living, partial hospitalization, and outpatient settings), which adds to the complexity.

Specific complication factors relevant to behavioral health care organizations include the following:

- The often-used team approach to behavioral health care makes consensus on diagnosis and treatment plans more difficult to achieve.
- A similar lack of consensus makes definition of achievable outcomes and outcomes evaluation difficult.
- The chronicity of some mental illnesses requires treatment goals that often are ameliorative, rather than curative, adding to the difficulty of measuring outcomes.
- The tracking of clients receiving multiple types of service, from multiple practitioners in multiple settings, is difficult.
- Information management systems may be less developed for behavioral health care services than for other health care sectors, making it difficult to identify relationships between care, cost, and care outcomes.
- Many important, high-volume clinical activities, such as "milieu" treatment, psychotherapy, and psychoeducational processes, are difficult to quantify and measure.
- Many factors in addition to treatment may influence the course of clinical activities.

To meet this challenge, behavioral health care organizations must improve quality and service outcomes, use resources efficiently, and satisfy internal/external customers. This framework is designed to help organizations pursue the goal of achieving optimal care outcomes at the lowest possible cost, using the appropriate level and amount of service.

Nine Dimensions of Performance

There are nine important dimensions of performance that affect the quality of outcomes and resource use. The dimensions are divided into two groups that comprise a traditional definition of quality: 1) Was the right thing done? and 2) Was it done right? One advantage of using the dimensions of performance is that they can be measured and improved, allowing an organization to track its progress. The nine dimensions of performance are efficacy, appropriateness, availability, timeliness, effectiveness, continuity, safety, efficiency, and respect and caring. These dimensions are defined in Table 1–1, pages 10–11.

Functions and Processes

The degree to which care fulfills the nine dimensions of performance is strongly influenced by the design and operation of a series of important clinical and organization functions. These functions include direct care activities (such as assessment, treatment, and education), as well as governance, management, and support services (such as information management and human resources management).

A *function* is defined as a group of processes with a common goal. A *process* is defined as a series of linked, goal-directed activities. For example, information management could be viewed as a function and data entry as a process within that function. Similarly, medication use could be viewed as a function and medication administration and clinical monitoring as processes within that function.

The processes involved in providing care and services to individuals in organizations are never isolated tasks, but are a series of activities that form important functions. The framework uses this important idea and focuses

Table 1–1 ■ Nine Dimensions of Performance

Doing the Right Thing

- The *efficacy* of the procedure or treatment in relation to the client's condition.
  The degree to which the care for the client has been shown to accomplish the desired/projected outcome(s).

- The *appropriateness* of a specific test, procedure, or service to meet the client's needs.
  The degree to which the care provided is relevant to the client's clinical needs, given the current state of knowledge.

Doing the Right Thing Well

- The *availability* of a needed test, procedure, treatment, or service to the client who needs it.
  The degree to which appropriate care is available to meet the client's needs.

- The *timeliness* with which a needed test, procedure, treatment, or service is provided to the client.
  The degree to which the care is provided to the client at the most beneficial or necessary time.

- The *effectiveness* with which tests, procedures, treatments, and services are provided.
  The degree to which the care is provided to the client at the most beneficial or necessary time.

- The *continuity* of the services provided to the client with respect to other services, clinicians, and providers, and over time.
  The degree to which the care for the client is coordinated among clinicians, among organizations, and across time.

- The *safety* of the client (and others) to whom the services are provided.
  The degree to which the risk of an intervention and risk in the care environment are reduced for the client and others, including providers.

- The *efficiency* with which services are provided.
  The relationship between the outcomes (results of care) and the resources used to deliver care.

Table 1–1 ■ Nine Dimensions of Performance (continued)

■ The *respect* and *caring* with which services are provided.
   The degree to which a client or designee is involved in his or her own
   care decisions, and to which those providing services do so with
   sensitivity and respect for the client's needs, expectations, and
   individual differences.

on the design, measurement, assessment, and improvement of functions as
well as of the processes within them. It is important to note that the
framework is not limited to improvement of direct care functions, but
clearly recognizes that governance, management, and support functions also
significantly influence care outcomes.

The Joint Commission's standards* are divided into two major
sections: individual-focused functions, which primarily involve direct and
indirect care to the individual, and organization-focused functions, which
do not involve direct care to the individual (see Table 1–2, page 12). This
focus on improving organization performance through attention to
processes and functions has several important implications. These implications underlie most of the activities described in this book and include the
following:

Effective care must cross organization boundaries. Most work in
behavioral health care organizations is accomplished by teams of inter-
dependent staff, whose individual efforts must be well coordinated to achieve
common goals. These goals cannot be accomplished unless processes and
communication can freely cross intra-organization boundaries; therefore,
different disciplines and different levels of staff must be able to
communicate and work together effectively. A corollary of the principle of
effective cross-communication is that in any specific design or improvement

---

* Refer to your most recent copy of the Joint Commission's *Accreditation Manual for
   Mental Health, Chemical Dependency, and Mental Retardation/Developmental Disabilities
   Services.*

Table 1–2 ■ Important Functions

Individual-focused Functions	Organization Functions
■ Rights, Responsibilities, and Ethics	■ Improving Organization Performance
■ Assessment	■ Leadership
■ Care, Treatment, and Service	■ Management of the Environment of Care
■ Education	■ Management of Human Resources
■ Continuum of Care	■ Management of Information
	■ Surveillance, Prevention, and Control of Infection

effort, one discipline alone will not be able to successfully implement a process that involves several disciplines.

In many behavioral health care organizations, the concept of teamwork is inherent in the philosophy of care. Much care in behavioral health settings is delivered using an interdisciplinary team. Members of a team may include psychiatrists and other physicians, clinical psychologists, psychiatric nurses, social workers, case managers, counselors and aides, substance abuse workers, support personnel, and volunteers. Other team members, such as a pharmacist, dietitian, certified academic teacher, physical therapist, or recreation therapist, may be added as needed in order to provide additional services to the individual being served. As the treatment team grows in number of members and complexity, the need for cross-discipline collaboration is greatly heightened.

Customer-supplier relationships need to be understood. Work is completed by enacting a series of customer-supplier relationships. Well-designed processes facilitate these transactions effectively. Additionally, all organizations have both internal customers and suppliers (for example, pharmacists and nurses in a clinical drug monitoring and administration process), and external customers (for example, major employers, payers, health plans) and suppliers (for example, special education resources in local public schools, food catering and vendors, computer software suppliers). A critical first step in improving organization performance is defining and identifying these customer-supplier relationships and their associated work processes. Once defined, these relationships must also be evaluated on a regular basis.

Outcomes must be defined and measured. Every process, by definition, produces results. Results may be intended and desirable, intended and undesirable, unintended and desirable, or unintended and undesirable. To determine how a process is performing, an organization can measure the activities involved in the process, but also, when possible, its outcomes. As noted earlier, care outcomes in behavioral health are likely to be more difficult to define and measure. Some likely outcomes dimensions include clinical status measures, physiologic-biochemical states, physical/functional capacity, psychological/psychosocial functioning, and family and work functioning. Integrative and evaluative outcomes should also be considered, including cost and satisfaction. (Refer to Appendix A, "A Primer on Behavioral Health Outcomes Measures," page 153, for more information.)

Variation in processes and outcomes should be analyzed. Some variation exists in all processes and, therefore, variability in their outcomes is normal. Analyzing the causes of and relative sizes of variation helps distinguish between a special cause (nonrecurring event) and a common or systemic cause. Analysis of variation and the knowledge gained from this study is an effective means of improving the performance of functions and processes.

Focus on improving processes rather than on individual performance. Ordinarily, designing or improving a process to achieve performance goals is best accomplished by focusing on the process, rather than on the individuals who carry it out. Both W. Edwards Deming and Joseph M. Juran, quality improvement leaders, demonstrated that in many instances the variation in outputs may be attributed to the effect of multiple causes in a system of common cause variation, rather than attributed to individual workers. Occasionally an individual's lack of knowledge, skill, sound judgment, or motivation will result in undesirable performance. Most major improvement opportunities, however, reside in processes.

Outcomes, Cost, Quality, and Value

The effect of an organization's performance of important functions can influence the

- quality of care;
- cost of its services;
- satisfaction of the individuals served and their family members;
- outcomes and the way they were achieved; and
- judgments important customers, including those individuals served, make about the quality and value of the care or service provided.

The framework described in this book focuses on improving the results of behavioral health care (including care outcomes) and on making better judgments about the quality and value of care.

Improving Performance

The framework for improving performance draws on the most successful approaches to improvement in health care and business, and combines these approaches into a logical and flexible cycle to carry out a wide range of improvement activities. As noted on page 13, these approaches all assume that significant opportunities for improvement will be found in designing and implementing organization functions and processes, rather than in scrutinizing an individual's performance. The key to improving performance (for example, outcomes, satisfaction, quality, value) is in systematically designing, measuring, assessing, and improving the organization's functions and processes.

▣ Components of the Framework for Improving Performance

The framework for improving performance reflects what an organization committed to excellence must minimally address. This framework is not limited to one method of improvement, nor is it limited just to improving performance. It recognizes that both external issues (such as health care reform and community needs) and internal issues (such as leadership and human resources) affect a behavioral health care organization's performance. Finally, it presents an adaptable cycle for designing, measuring, assessing, and improving processes and outcomes in a behavioral health care organization.

Figure 1–1, page 16, illustrates this framework's three basic components:

- External environment;
- Internal environment; and
- Cycle for improving performance.

External Environment

Factors outside a behavioral health care organization significantly affect the way the organization designs and carries out its services (see Table 1–3, page 17). Organizations must recognize how such factors in the external environment affect the organization's internal environment, organization priorities, and performance improvement efforts. To stay in a proactive position, organizations should continuously survey their environment, elicit feedback from customers and others, and act accordingly. Today, behavioral health care organizations must monitor and address at least the following external forces:

Health care reform. The need to prepare for and respond to ongoing and major reconfigurations in the health care delivery and payment system.

Purchasers. The need to address the expectations of purchasers (for example, HMOs, POSs, PPOs, case management, insurers).

The Joint Commission. The need to meet nationally recognized standards.

Regulators. The need to fulfill state and federal regulatory requirements, which affect the design of many services.

Accountability. The need to demonstrate to others (including the individuals being served, the community, and purchasers) the quality and value of the care provided.

Framework for Improving Performance

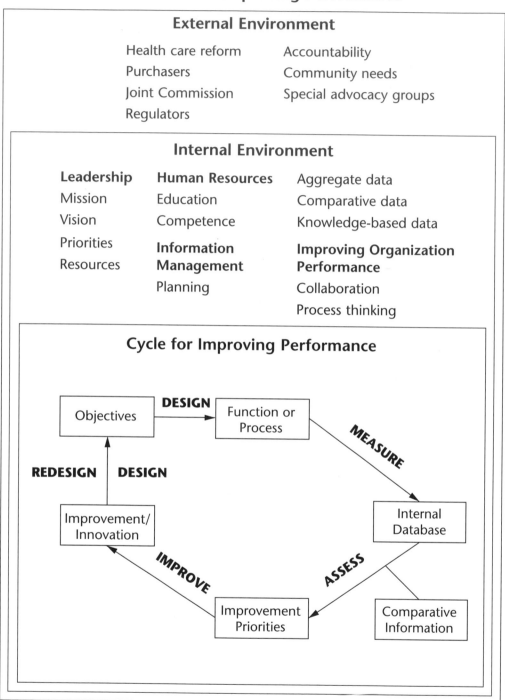

Figure 1–1 ■ *This illustration depicts the three core components of the framework for improving performance: external environment, internal environment, and cycle for improving performance.*

Table 1–3 ■ Framework for Improving Performance— External Environment

External Environment

- Health care reform
- Purchasers
- Joint Commission
- Regulators

- Accountability
- Community needs
- Special advocacy groups

Community needs. The need to understand and address the needs and expectations of the community served.

Special advocacy groups. The need to recognize and form collaborative working relationships with groups developed to advance rights and concerns of individuals served.

Consumers are most interested in

- safe and effective services,
- fair access to service,
- cost effectiveness,
- the empowerment of consumers through education and board representation, and
- fair representation of alternative services.

Internal Environment

The internal environment—the second component of this framework—is a blanket term for the many functions existing inside an organization that most influence performance, including efforts to design, measure, assess, and improve processes (see Table 1–4, page 18). The following internal functions are most important in determining the overall quality and value of the care and other services provided by a behavioral health care organization:

- Leadership,
- Human resource management,
- Information management, and
- Improving organization performance.

Table 1–4 ■ Framework for Improving Performance—Internal Environment

Leadership

- Mission
- Vision
- Priorities
- Resources

Human Resources Management

- Education
- Competence

Information Management

- Planning
- Aggregate data
- Comparative data
- Knowledge-based data

Improving Organization Performance

- Collaboration
- Process thinking

Leadership. Leaders in an organization typically include the members of the governing body, the chief executive officer, the clinical director, the discipline chief, the unit or service director, and other senior managers. In small behavioral health care organizations, one individual may serve in more than one of these leadership roles. The internal environment is significantly shaped by the leadership of the organization.

Effective leaders share certain qualities, including

- expertise in their areas of responsibility;
- knowledge about improvement, including an understanding of systems, variation, measurement, and the psychology of human behavior and motivation;

- authority and willingness to allocate resources for improvement activities;
- an understanding that continuous improvement is essential to an organization's success;
- a passion for improvement;
- an understanding of organizations and of organization change; and
- vision.

One crucial responsibility for leaders is organization planning. Leaders, with members of the organization, must define strategic plans that are consistent with the organization's mission and vision. Once developed, the leaders must communicate these plans throughout the organization and allocate resources for their accomplishment. The Joint Commission's leadership standards* require that the strategic plan set the organization's priorities for performance improvement and be aligned with the organization's mission and identified community needs. This is an enormously important activity, given the scarcity of resources and growing cost-containment forces.

Other leadership activities can also have great influence on an organization's performance. For example, building teamwork and fostering continuous improvement often require leaders to become better facilitators and coaches. (Refer to Appendix B, "Optimizing Teams and Teamwork," page 167, for more information.) In this role, they encourage constant learning, innovation, and risk taking. Similarly, empowerment is a concept gaining support and commitment among leaders and considered essential for successful leadership. Many effective leaders empower staff throughout the organization to acquire and apply the knowledge and skills to continuously improve processes and services. Leaders also encourage continuous

---

* Refer to your most recent copy of the Joint Commission's *Accreditation Manual for Mental Health, Chemical Dependency, and Mental Retardation/Developmental Disabilities Services.*

improvement through their personal and direct involvement in measurement, assessment, and improvement activities—especially as they apply to the leadership process itself.

Human resources management. An organization must have an adequate number of competent clinical and support staff, including volunteers, if applicable, available to carry out all key governance, management, clinical, and support processes to fulfill its objectives, including continuous improvement efforts. As in all personnel management areas, staff performance must be regularly assessed and improved through continuing education and training opportunities. Continuous feedback of performance of critical functions is essential for quality improvement.

Information management. Quality care depends on timely, valid, and reliable information about

- the science of health care delivery, including behavioral health services, both separately and as components in the continuum of care services;
- the individual being served, his or her care, and treatment results;
- management and business functions;
- performance of the organization as a whole;
- other organizations' performance from external reference databases, if available; and
- knowledge of emerging clinical pathways and best practices.

It is essential that an organization meet these information needs to coordinate, integrate, assess, and improve services.

Improving organization performance. Organizations that excel evaluate themselves rigorously and strive to improve. These organizations are balanced between the demands of everyday functions (for example, arranging crisis admissions and staffing plans for the day) and the need for continuous organization improvement. With forethought, organizations can create well-designed processes, measure the performance of existing processes, assess processes based on measurement data, and improve outcomes by redesigning existing processes or by designing new processes when necessary. The Joint Commission's improving organization performance standards* are compatible with a variety of process improvement methodologies. Many of these methodologies share key concepts that are common to almost all performance improvement approaches:

- *Assessment of customer satisfaction and experience.* It is essential to consider the individual served and others' judgments about quality, their view of the need for improvement, and their experience with care delivery.
- *Technology and environment of care measurement.* It is important to ensure that processes are in place to evaluate the equipment, machinery, and supplies used in care delivery.
- *Research and knowledge building.* An organization must continually search for better and more efficient ways to perform functions and processes.
- *Systematic performance improvement.* Close coordination and collaboration are necessary among organization units (for example, clinical, customer service, billing, data entry, or clerical staff), services, and disciplines.
- *Process focus.* Improvement opportunities usually lie in processes, not in an individual clinical staff's performance.

It is important to note that these approaches begin with the assumption that the majority of clinical staff are intrinsically motivated to perform well

---

* Refer to your most recent copy of the Joint Commission's *Accreditation Manual for Mental Health, Chemical Dependency, and Mental Retardation/Developmental Disabilities Services.*

and genuinely desire to help their organization achieve its goals. This philosophy contrasts sharply with the sometimes punitive connotations often associated with earlier quality assurance efforts.

Cycle for Improving Performance

An organization must have a systematic approach to improvement. The cycle for improving performance—the third component of this framework—describes such an approach. This cycle is anchored in the real work of an organization—the functions and processes it carries out every day to pursue its goals and mission. This cycle can be carried out by existing work groups as part of everyday activities.

When the processes or functions being addressed cross service, discipline, or department boundaries, it is especially helpful to form a representative team composed of the people who have ownership of the process, who are responsible for the process, who carry out the process, and who are affected by the process. Cross-functional and cross-discipline processes are considered especially important because they are often the basis of improving organization performance in behavioral health care organizations.

To improve processes and outcomes over time, staff (working from a known set of objectives and mission) must systematically and scientifically design, measure, assess, and improve these processes and outcomes.

Figure 1–2, page 23, describes the building blocks of the improvement cycle. As its cyclical nature suggests, improvement work can begin at any point in the cycle. Specific tenets of the cycle include the following:

- *Objectives* for achieving a clear goal or purpose are necessary before launching a design effort.
- A design effort results in a *function or process*—that is, a related series of activities directed toward accomplishing a specific goal.
- Measuring performance of a function or process results in an *internal database,* which is used to establish baseline data and to assess performance over time.

Cycle for Improving Performance

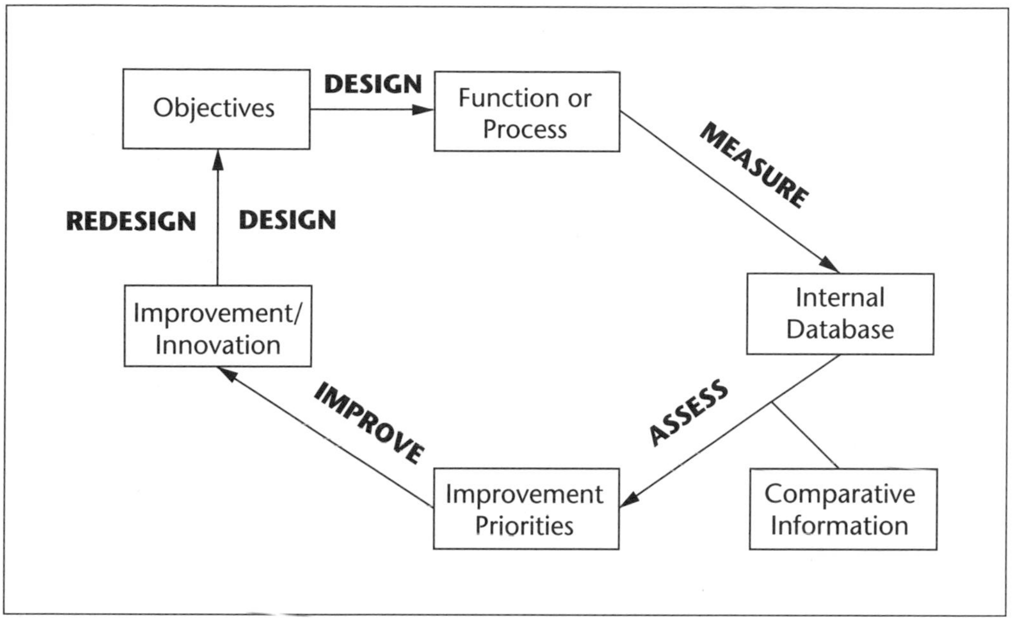

Figure 1–2 ■ *This cycle is composed of activities (represented by the arrows) and their related inputs and outputs (in boxes). The cycle can be entered at any point.*

- One of the tools used to assess performance is *comparative information* from other sources, such as reference databases, practice guidelines, and best practices.
- Assessment of a process should result in identifying *opportunities for improvement* and setting *priorities*.
- Based on these priorities, the organization creates, tests, and implements specific *improvements and innovations,* which involve redesign or a new design, respectively, of a process or function.

It is important to note that the cycle continues even after it has been completed for a given function or process for the first time. The objectives are viewed, reviewed, and perhaps changed again; new information is captured from a similar facility using a similar process. Simultaneously, measurement continues in order to determine whether improvement has occurred and can be sustained, and the internal database continues to grow.

Assessment and evaluation using cumulative information may identify further opportunities for improvement.

The improvement cycle is truly a model for understanding organization change. Hence, it may be applied at any level of generality or specificity. For example, *function* could refer to the entire behavioral health care organization as a system (either freestanding or as part of a complex behavioral health care system or multi-office national organization), or it could refer to a multidisciplinary, cross-service activity (such as client assessment or interdisciplinary team care planning). *Process* could refer to a number of activities (for example, how family members are instructed to care for their attention-deficit/hyperactive child, how eating-disordered adolescents are instructed on their diet and medications, how preventive maintenance for basic life safety is managed for an older individual with features associated with dementia in a residential care program). Process may also refer to support and managerial tasks (for example, how a case manager reviews each individual's status biweekly in a CMHC with particular reference to housing, medication stabilization, and nutrition).

Subsequent chapters of this book provide more in-depth explanation of these concepts and improvement appraisals and specific examples of how to carry out this cycle.

Relationship of the Cycle to the Joint Commission's Standards*

The cycle for improving organization performance is the basis of the Joint Commission's improving organization performance standards. Please refer to these standards, intent statements, and scoring guidelines. The standards, like the cycle, focus primarily on the performance of an organization's systems and processes, not solely on performance of individuals.

---

* Refer to your most recent copy of the Joint Commission's *Accreditation Manual for Mental Health, Chemical Dependency, and Mental Retardation/Developmental Disabilities Services.*

▣ Chapter Summary

Underlying Principles

- The purpose of behavioral health care is to maximize an individual's health and to use resources efficiently and appropriately.

- Care outcomes and use of resources are affected by the nine measurable dimensions of performance: efficacy, appropriateness, availability, timeliness, effectiveness, continuity, safety, efficiency, and respect and caring.

- The degree to which behavioral health care organizations fulfill these nine dimensions of performance is strongly influenced by the design and operation of a series of important functions and processes.

- Leadership and collaboration are essential for behavioral health care professionals, especially in the current health care environment.

- The effect of an organization's performance of its important functions is evident in care outcomes, in satisfaction with its services, in the cost of its services, and in the judgments about the quality and value of these services made by the organization and others.

Components of the Framework for Improving Performance

The framework incorporates the best ideas and methods into a flexible approach to improvement. The framework has three basic components:

- External environment;
- Internal environment; and
- Cycle for improving performance.

2

Design

design (di-'zTn), v.t. to draw, mark, or plan out; project; set apart mentally: v.i. to formulate designs or execute original work: n. an outline, plan, or drawing; project; intention.

—*Webster's New School and Office Dictionary*

- Why Do We Design? Setting Objectives
- What Do We Design? Functions and Processes
- How Do We Design?
- Who Creates the Design?
- Examples of Design
- Chapter Summary

Conducting a psychosocial assessment and intervention with an individual . . . calling a chemical dependency individual to schedule a family visit . . . creating an interdisciplinary treatment plan for a psychiatric inpatient and his or her family . . . implementing a behavioral plan for a developmentally delayed child . . . implementing a computerized information system. No single activity, process, or function in a behavioral health care organization is an end in itself, but each is a necessary component of a larger whole. Each activity is designed to fulfill a specific objective and is carefully interwoven into the organization structure.

When reviewing the organization, office, branch, department, program, service, team, or individual level of performance, behavioral health care professionals need to regularly stop and ask themselves two vital questions:

- What goals are we trying to accomplish?
- How can we best accomplish those goals?

These questions are the essence of the design concept. The design component of the cycle for improving performance focuses on determining specific objectives of an organization's activities, and developing, designing, and implementing functions and processes to achieve those objectives.

As behavioral health care organizations attempt to better serve their customers and stay competitive, many are designing and offering new services or are redesigning their present services to be more efficient, to be more user friendly, and to produce better care outcomes. Some organizations' processes and functions reflect local policy, or are a response to regulatory pressure or administrative directives, rather than following a carefully integrative design.

Figure 2–1, page 29, illustrates how design fits into the cycle for improving performance. As noted earlier, one component of the cycle does not have to be completed before another is begun. The inputs for design are organization objectives; leaders must decide what they want the new design to accomplish. Design activities can involve multiple phases, each of which may include some measurement and benchmarking to ensure that the project is proceeding as planned, and, if it's not, appropriate modifications should be made.

Many of the same techniques apply to designing a new process and redesigning an existing process. However, it is important to distinguish between *design* and *redesign*. *Design* creates new processes—in effect, starting with a clean slate. *Redesign* takes a fresh look at an existing process—in effect, revising and improving the process. For example, to redesign a process, an organization would most likely use information about its current performance of the process as part of the effort. An

Cycle for Improving Performance—Design

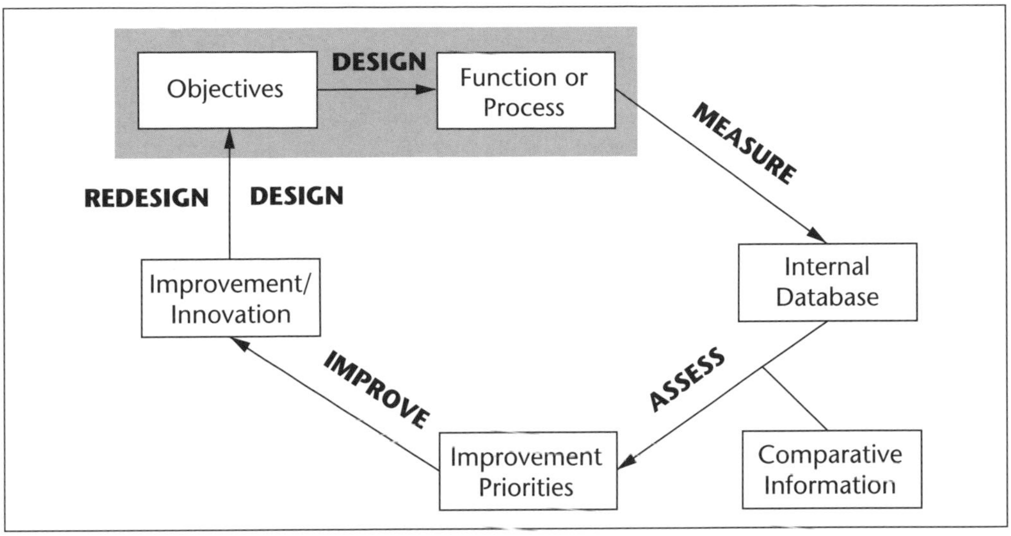

Figure 2–1 ■ *This figure highlights the **design** stage of the improvement cycle—the subject of this chapter.*

organization creating a new design would not have that information to use, because the process would not yet exist. Both design and redesign can be very helpful in driving improvement efforts and many of the same techniques apply to both (for example, reviewing state-of-the-art knowledge about the process).

This chapter focuses primarily on design of new activities. It is intended for organizations that may be, for example, opening a therapeutic foster care/supportive living service in a new community, extending a product line (such as developing a "walk in" assessment for crisis intervention), or offering new clinical services (such as a dual diagnosis group for individuals with chemical dependency and mental health problems).

▣ Why Do We Design? Setting Objectives

Organization objectives and organization process are intrinsically tied together through design. To be successful in this process, an organization must set goals related to its mission, vision, and other plans.

Organization processes should reflect these goals. Unfortunately, in many contemporary health care organizations, the objectives of a process are often unexpressed (unwritten and unspoken), resulting in less effective work processes. When approaching the concept of design, all activities should be regularly examined for their relevance, value, feasibility, and effectiveness.

Such an examination, which may be accomplished using existing everyday work tasks (for example, preparing an individual for admission or discharge), may lead an organization's leaders to conclude that a new process is needed or that an existing process needs to be redesigned. Therefore, organizations should have a systematic process in place for

- reviewing organization goals and the activities that fulfill them;
- reviewing and selecting opportunities that require a new design effort;
- designing new processes or functions; and
- measuring and assessing the new processes or functions.

This systematic process helps an organization identify opportunities for innovation. It provides a method to fairly weigh the benefits and drawbacks of a newly designed process or function. It also provides a method to involve the right people at the start and get the best knowledge for creating the design. Finally, it determines whether the results of the design effort meet the objectives.

Organization goals are not created in isolation. Development of an organization's goals and the design of activities to pursue those goals require an organization to ask the following questions:

- Is this process, function, or service consistent with the organization's mission, vision, and other plans?
- What do the organization's clients, staff, and other customers expect from the process, function, or service, and how do they think it should work?

- What do scientific and professional experts and other reliable sources say about the design process or function?
- What information is available about the performance of similar processes, functions, or services in other organizations?

The answers to these questions help the organization develop a basic set of performance expectations that guide process design, as well as measurement and assessment of the process, function, or service.

Mission, Vision, and Plans

Any design should consider how the resulting process or function will serve the organization's

- mission,
- future vision, and
- plans for carrying out its mission and fulfilling its vision.

The organization's mission, vision, and plans answer the basic question "What is the organization for?" One of the best methods to define an organization's work is in relation to its primary activities. An environmental assessment is also an important source of information used to establish mission, vision, and plans, and analyzes whether current activities are fulfilling an organization's overall strategic plan. Such data help leaders determine how the vision of the organization (in the future) will serve the community. For example, it may reveal that in a specific community, support services to single-parent families are insufficient to meet the needs of this rapidly growing population segment or that home-based behavioral health services need to expand to meet existing needs. These elements (mission, vision, and plans) are also important for the organization to develop a shared sense of identity and culture.

Needs, Expectations, and Experiences of Individuals Served, Staff, and Others

To design successful processes and functions yielding better outcomes, behavioral health care organizations must understand the needs, expectations, and experiences of individuals served and their families.

A comprehensive community-based needs assessment has been a tenet of behavioral health care practice for years. The individuals served and their families are the primary consumers of the behavioral health care services. Meeting their needs is critical to an organization's survival. Once these needs, expectations, and experiences are understood, the organization can decide how and to what extent they can be met.

Equally important are the internal customers—the organization's clinical and support staff, and volunteers who will carry out processes. Organization goals must take into account their needs and expectations. Understanding the perspective of internal customers can be quite powerful, and can help all staff work in a collaborative manner and become more attuned to each other's needs and expectations. Other important customers and suppliers to consider in this process are purchasers, payers, physicians, referral sources, accreditors, regulators, and the community as a whole.

Discussing the nine dimensions of performance (efficacy, appropriateness, availability, timeliness, effectiveness, continuity, safety, efficiency, and respect and caring) (refer to page 9) with specific groups is an excellent way to elicit needs and expectations. This can be accomplished using focus groups or sampling from existing committees or advisory groups. As the data become available, measures can be established to determine if the services provided fulfill the needs and expectations within the dimensions of performance.

Current Knowledge About Organization and Clinical Activities

Improvement requires knowledge. An organization's goals—and any activities designed to pursue those goals—must consider the best knowledge available concerning management and clinical activities. If, for example, an organization wants to change its scheduling hours during which care is available, or the scope and frequency of psychosocial support groups, it should consider both current practices within the organization and other existing state-of-the-art practices. Such knowledge is available from expert sources both inside and outside an organization, including other behavioral health care organizations, other health care organizations with similar processes, professional literature, professional societies, trade associations, and consultants.

Likewise, expert knowledge of current practices is crucial in the design of any clinical or individual-focused care activities. Contemporary clinical knowledge can be found in information on clinical pathways, parameters of care, scientific and research literature, practice guidelines, and standards of care. Several examples throughout this book show behavioral health care organizations using subject matter expertise as a tool for successful design and improvement. Over time, the rapid development of health knowledge databases will be specifically designed and more readily available for these purposes.

Relevant Data

Data are the cornerstone of successful design and improvement efforts. The importance of valid, reliable data and the effective use of these data cannot be overemphasized. For example, a behavioral health care organization would not decide to introduce a therapeutic foster care program without knowledge about the client volume's relationship to current residential occupancy levels, foster parent staffing, academic needs, community acceptance, and so on.

For redesign and other improvement efforts, information about care outcomes is especially valuable. Outcomes data should encompass both specific performance within the organization (for example, aggregate data showing historical rates of specific outcomes for specific diagnoses) and information from existing reference databases (for example, average time and frequency of relapse after drug and alcohol residential treatment). Information from reference databases (compiled by professional or trade associations, behavioral health care systems, payers, regulatory agencies, accreditation agencies, and others) can help organizations determine their goals for the individual served and organization outcomes. Existing health services research information is an added resource in this area. Use of aggregate and summary data in performance improvement efforts is described in more detail in Chapter 3, page 65.

Availability of Resources

In the current climate, behavioral health organizations are painfully aware that their resources are limited. Limited financial resources have affected many areas, including clinical staffing levels, in clients' expected length of stay, residential occupancies, and staff quality. Funding cuts have also spawned innovative treatment approaches, such as home-based psychiatric care.

Every organization seeks ways to control costs and improve efficiency without sacrificing quality or essential services. In their short-range and long-range planning, organizations face daunting decisions as they weigh their mission and vision against their resources. Organizations contemplating new design efforts must weigh the availability of resources against the potential benefits for the individual and for the organization. Ideally, quality planning and business planning can be integrated to provide cost/benefit analysis for critical decisions. The visionary leader's dreams and the operations manager's pragmatism need to be reconciled with current resources.

▣ What Do We Design? Functions and Processes

When addressing what to design, think in terms of the everyday work of behavioral health care organizations. This work can be defined in terms of numerous functions and processes. Stated another way, what is actually created, made, produced, conducted by the organization?

As described in Chapter 1, page 9, a function is a group of processes with a common goal. A process is a series of linked, goal-directed activities. For example, *function* could refer to an activity of the organization as a system. This system may be a freestanding community-based organization or part of a larger health system or multi-site national care provider. Function could also refer to a multidisciplinary, cross-service activity (for example, assessment, care treatment, medication monitoring, education).

A process can be a clinical activity. For example, *process* can also refer to the systematic way that chemical dependency counselors assess the history of addiction and an individual's psychosocial experiences and other symptoms. Or, it could refer to the specific steps for discharge planning or the steps in preparation for a referral to support groups and residential/supportive living. It could also refer to how cases in an outpatient behavioral health care clinic are scheduled and how the continuum of care is received and assigned.

▣ How Do We Design?

Any new process design must pay careful attention to the customer-supplier relationships inherent in the process. The design should facilitate the greatest efficiency in these relationships, coordinating and integrating all relevant activities to produce desirable outcomes.

To create a new design for care delivery, management, or support processes, organizations should consider the following process design guidelines:

- *Design a systematic method to determine the process' effect on the organization's mission, vision, plans, customers, resources, and so forth.* Surveys, informal discussions, focus groups, and consensus techniques are useful tools.

- *Base decisions on valid, reliable data.* Data are key to developing accurate design specifications and to assessing the effectiveness of the design.

- *Involve the right people.* Any design effort should include representatives of all groups who are responsible for and participate in the process, including the individuals served (that is, all process owners).

- *Strategically review a variety of information on the subject.* Examine the professional literature, advice of professional societies or trade associations, and practices of other organizations. A view of other organizations' practices and experiences can also help prevent mistakes early on and can inspire creative thinking.

Several key additional building blocks relevant to the design process include the following:

- Understand client needs, expectations, and preferences;
- Review the type and nature of care delivered; and
- Be knowledgeable of the organization's design, structure, and work processes.

▣ Who Creates the Design?

All staff participate in the design process. The Joint Commission's leadership standards* require that leaders and managers take a special and active role in overseeing and setting priorities for design. Generally, managers are responsible for processes within their areas; design of processes with a wider scope may be overseen by upper management or by a team of managers.

Design and redesign efforts require resources. Leaders must ensure that the staff involved have the necessary resources and expertise to accomplish their task. Further, their authority to make changes should be commensurate with their responsibility for process improvements. Although regular feedback and contact with management are important, rigid control can stifle creativity. A good balance of guidance and direction with ample freedom and systematic feedback is indicated.

The group that creates the process should include the people responsible for the process, the staff who will carry out the process, and the staff affected by the process. As appropriate, the group members could include staff from different services, different disciplines, and different job categories. When the group needs a perspective not offered by its representatives, it should conduct interviews or surveys outside the group or invite new members into the work group.

---

* Refer to your most recent copy of the Joint Commission's *Accreditation Manual for Mental Health, Chemical Dependency, and Mental Retardation/Developmental Disabilities Services*.

Examples of Design

◎ Example 2-1: Accessibility to Care: A TQM/CQI Application in a Behavioral Health and Chemical Dependency Setting

Note: This case study illustrates practical and real world first-stage applications of TQM/CQI in psychiatric and chemical dependency settings. It is important to note that the framework for improving performance is not dependent on the principles of TQM/CQI; however, it is completely compatible with these and other improvement methodology principles and theories. This case study highlights how the problem was identified, the leadership support and project data collection and outcome, and ongoing performance monitoring.

The Setting and Background

The setting is a large community mental health center (CMHC) that has merged with a large acute care hospital and is part of a larger comprehensive health care system. The CMHC offers a full continuum of care, including inpatient and emergency psychiatric service, traditional outpatient programs, partial and continuing treatment programs, and a variety of prevention and psychoeducational services. The facility was attempting to balance an increasing demand from the community, cost-cutting and cost-containment forces from the state and other regulatory agencies, and increasing difficulty with services accessibility. The CMHC has approximately 4,000 individuals enrolled in active care at any given time.

The Problem

The broad problem of accessibility included referral patterns, triage and client routing, decision making involving levels of care and continuum of care step-downs, and meeting the day-to-day demands on the treatment system. More specifically, the accessibility problem appeared in the form of

- long waiting times to enter treatment,
- complicated referral forms and paperwork,
- frustration among behavioral health system and primary care providers attempting to refer clients to care, and
- ultimately lost opportunities to provide care and lost revenues.

The problem was first reviewed by the management and administrative group in the behavioral health care center and a project team was launched with the approval of the health system's total quality management (TQM) oversight committee.

The Project Team

The project team was composed of clinicians, managers, administrators, program coordinators, and front-line clinicians. The members included a mix of employees from various professional backgrounds, including nursing, psychology, social work, and psychiatric rehabilitation. Team members were selected from volunteers and staff who had a vital interest in the problem (such as, team coordinators). There were 11 team members, but attendance varied from meeting to meeting, with a core group of eight members. Approximately half of the team members were formally trained in TQM/continuous quality improvement (CQI) methods. This inconsistent training proved to be a barrier as significant time was spent explaining terms, bringing other clinicians up to speed with regard to TQM/CQI methods, and teaching TQM/CQI tools rather than addressing the problem during early project team meetings. The project team met on a weekly basis for eight months, with several half-day retreats to allow for a more intensive working phase.

The Process

Defining the problem. The team began with a very global and wide-ranging discussion of access to internal programs and external services. It also discussed concepts concerning the organization and the existing structure of programs as related to mandated changes with managed care, the need for immediate access to care for crisis situations (for example, partial hospitalization), and state regulatory influences. The group began with a brainstorming session on central issues regarding hindrances to client movement within the system. This discussion yielded a long list of reasons, including

- poor internal communication,
- backlogs of clients,
- insurance and managed care forces,
- state and federal regulations,
- loss of acute inpatient psychiatric beds in the large community,
- lack of integrated clinical identity,
- lack of flexibility and adaptability within clinical screening teams,

- lack of access to information and centralized record keeping,
- complicated paperwork,
- staff turnover and staff shortage,
- limited time and resources,
- unclear criteria for levels of care,
- lack of information for clients and their families, and
- lack of community support and a unified mission.

Solidifying the team. As the team progressed, additional members were added who could more adequately represent various care areas, particularly those service areas where triage and disposition of clients were of critical importance (such as the psychiatric emergency service). As the team process continued, ground rules were periodically reviewed to improve attendance and performance within the team, and to achieve maximum utilization of time and resources. The review of ground rules and team expectations was especially helpful, given the fact that all team members were still not formally trained in TQM methods.

First-round cause-and-effect diagram. Subsequent meetings began to further delineate problems in critical areas, including a more specific review of psychiatric inpatient, outpatient, and emergency services. These efforts were considered preliminary cause-and-effect diagrams, with an attempt to link causal factors identified in programs to actual care outcomes. (See page 103 for a detailed explanation of cause-and-effect diagrams.)

The group also spent a significant amount of time attempting to delineate, in a more precise way, the factors leading to difficult access within specified program areas. The project team periodically reviewed the key fundamental definitions of the "as is" and "desired state" statements for accessibility to make sure they were on the right track.

The desired state was identified as access to all levels of care for new, readmitted, and transferred clients that occurs in an efficient and expeditious manner. Using the list of reasons for hindrance of client movement identified in the brainstorming session, the team began to rank key areas of data collection based on these early causal hypotheses.

Using a cause-and-effect diagram with people, methods, machines, and material dimensions, the group refined its earlier brainstorming with an initial causal analysis. A large system cause-and-effect diagram was developed.

Pruning the cause-and-effect diagram. The original cause-and-effect diagram contained approximately 50 causal links. It was reduced to the modified diagram shown in Figure 2–2, page 42, which represented many important pathways and dimensions.

Further team meetings led to a more detailed cause-and-effect analysis for each dimension relevant to missed appointments. Figure 2–3, page 43, illustrates the more detailed diagram linking the treatment and illness characteristics, appointment procedures, and unexpected life events to the missed appointments for the "no shows" category. This cause-and-effect analysis was followed up with a data collection effort for each site and program, including information on location of service, client diagnosis, source of referral, waiting time to service, occurrence of contact with clinic prior to appointment, insurance status, number of previous no shows in the last year, transportation type, and reasons for missed appointments.

Benchmarking from a distance. The team also conducted a modest benchmarking effort and reviewed no show and lost appointment rates in their local community. In addition, a targeted literature review was conducted to look at existing research on the topics and potential solutions.

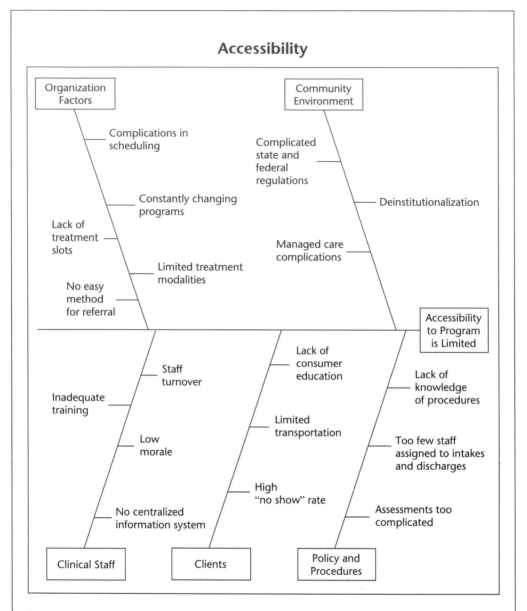

Figure 2–2 ■ *This cause-and-effect diagram illustrates the large number of possible causes of missed program accessibility.*

Data collection and analysis. Approximately 600 missed appointment cases were collected across the system. Number of previous no shows in last year, number of no shows by clinical site, reason for no

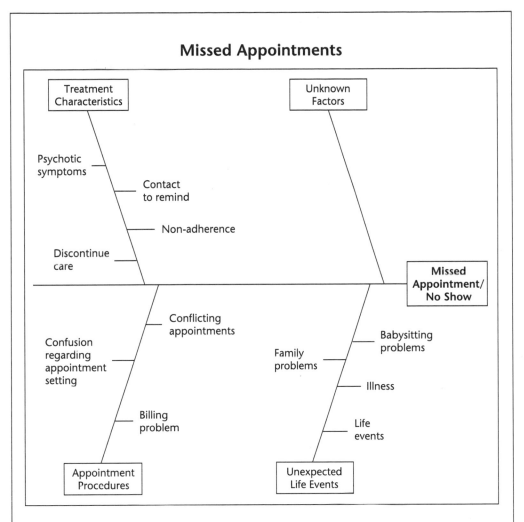

Figure 2–3 ■ *This cause-and-effect diagram illustrates the large number of possible causes of missed appointments.*

shows, associated correlations, and cross-tabulations were examined (refer to Figure 2–4, page 44).

Results and Outcomes

Using the cause-and-effect diagram, the team began a brainstorming session focused on important changes that might affect

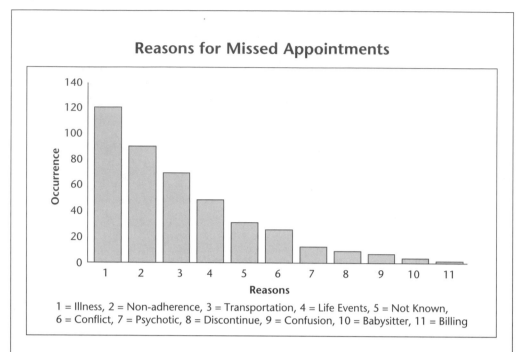

Figure 2–4 ■ *This Pareto chart depicts the frequency of reasons for missed appointments. (Refer to page 105 for a detailed explanation of Pareto charts.)*

accessibility within the system. A number of ideas were generated and reviewed; some were quickly implemented and tracked, including

- development of an adult crisis service,
- use of a more flexible and efficient appointment-setting procedure, and
- expansion of group therapy services.

Further detailed analysis was also conducted on the missed appointments including explanation of specific reasons, such as

- illness,
- client non-adherence,
- transportation, and
- other unexpected life events.

An analysis of no shows over the past year indicated that most clients missed from one to five appointments, but some missed many more, particularly in programs that offer services each day.

Analysis by clinical site suggested a significant interaction between each service, type of client, and nature of missed appointments. No relationship was seen by diagnosis, presence of Axis II psychopathology, and number of previous no shows. More chronic clients did, as expected, show a significantly higher no-show rate.

Finally, a strong relationship was identified between contact with clients prior to the scheduled appointment and no-show rates. This finding is reinforced by literature and data from community benchmarking. The reviewed information suggested that any contact with a client prior to the scheduled visit increased the likelihood of keeping the appointment. This was true for all programs except the children's clinic and a program for the seriously and persistently mentally ill, which involved intensive case management.

Additional positive outcomes were realized, including scheduling changes and the development of a new adult clinic. One of the most impressive outcomes was that the team was also able to shorten a five-week appointment wait to five days with these changes.

Continuous monitoring to track initial changes and to assess additional recommended improvements are underway. The team is now reviewing the viability of

- standardizing a client contact prior to each visit,
- developing local teams to further identify individual differences for missed appointments at each clinic site,
- using a more aggressive outreach procedure for the seriously and persistently mentally ill, and
- implementing an early "warning" detection system for awareness of client illness and transportation problems.

▣ **Example 2-2: Improving Dual Diagnosis Treatment in a Community Mental Health Center**

Note: This example illustrates how organizations can successfully design a process. In both this and the previous example, the organization selected the process only after carefully considering the effect on the organization's mission, vision, and plan, and on staff, clients, and other customers and suppliers. In both examples, the organizations formed teams of people important to the process. The teams collected data about needs and expectations, practices outside the organization, and resource implications to form the basis for the design and the implementation plan.

The Setting and Background

This CMHC offers a full continuum of care, with special interest in dual diagnosis clients. This particular community center is part of a large health system and has an independent service that offers treat-ment for chemical dependency.

The Problem

Since the health system has two separate entities, mental health and chemical dependency, it has historically struggled with clients who have dual diagnosis problems. Specifically, the problem appeared in the form of

- dual diagnosis clients receiving relatively poor care and often using the emergency room for service,
- a lack of clear coordination between the two service areas (that is, mental health and chemical dependency), and

- billing and revenue problems associated with exhaustion of care benefits by one of the service areas.

The Project Team

A project team was formed and consisted of clinicians, managers, administrators, and front-line triage staff. Many individuals who had ownership in the problem were also nominated for the team.

The Process

The team began its work at a very basic level. It conducted a literature review of incidence of dual diagnosis clients from two standpoints: prevalence of substance abuse disorders for clients seeking treatment for other psychiatric disorders and prevalence of coexisting psychiatric disorders in clients seeking primary substance abuse treatment. A consistency of findings emerged. From both sets of studies (see Table 2–1, page 48, and Table 2–2, page 49) a very high co-morbidity rate was reported, ranging from approximately 37% to 76% of clients presenting in either sector showing evidence of dual diagnosis symptoms.

Following the literature review, the team began to review general themes in the treatment of dual diagnosis clients, including parallel versus sequential treatment, care versus confrontation, abstinence-oriented versus abstinence-mandated programs (a particularly important difference between the separate treatment facilities' philosophies), and institutionalization versus recovery and rehabilitation. A conceptual consensus emerged in the team suggesting that the diagnosis and treatment of these clients is difficult, that the assessment of dual diagnosis clients requires a careful and systematic approach, and that an integrated theoretical and clinical framework would hold the best promise for effective treatment.

Table 2–1 ■ **Prevalence of Substance Use Disorders in Clients Seeking Treatment for Other Psychiatric Disorders**

Authors	Study Sample	Findings
McLellan and Druley	279 hospitalized psychiatric clients (60% schizophrenic, 30% depressed)	49% reported substance abuse problem
Drake and Wallach	187 chronically mentally ill (mostly schizophrenic clients in community)	25% abusing alcohol, 18% abusing drugs
Caton, et al	100 hospitalized psychiatric clients (37% depressed, 21% schizophrenic)	51% abusing substance; one-third of this group began substance abuse before onset of psychopathology
Miller, et al	110 hospitalized psychiatric clients (50 schizophrenic, 60 bipolar)	50% of schizophrenics, 25% of bipolar patients abused ≥ 1 drug

Source: Adopted from: Substance abuse and mental illness—the dually diagnosed patient. *The American Journal on Addictions* 1(2), 1992. Reprinted with permission.

In addition to the literature review and review of conceptual and clinical treatment approaches for these clients, a number of specific steps were undertaken. These steps included

- a field survey of staff experience,
- review of adverse incidents and client events,
- identification of all internal and external customers,
- tracking of client referrals inside and outside the facilities, and
- a review of the history of dual diagnosis treatment in the health system.

Table 2–2 ■ Prevalence of Coexisting Psychiatric Disorders in Clients Seeking Primary Substance Abuse Treatment

Authors	Study Sample	Findings
Ross, et al	501 clients (68% alcohol abusers, 32% drug abusers)	76% had another lifetime diagnosis, 65% had current diagnosis
Rounsavile, et al	298 cocaine addicts	74% had lifetime non-substance abuse diagnosis, 56% had current diagnosis
Khantzian and Treece	133 opioid addicts	77% had current Axis I diagnosis, 65% had Axis II diagnosis
Mirin, et al	350 drug abusers	37% had another Axis I diagnosis (currently ill plus previously ill when drug free)

Source: Adopted from: Substance abuse and mental illness—the dually diagnosed patient. *The American Journal on Addictions* 1(2), 1992. Reprinted with permission.

This last activity was very difficult and highlighted the logistical and clinical problems that exist in treating dual diagnosis clients in the system, particularly those problems related to adverse incidents, inappropriate triage in the emergency room, and higher care expenditures than would have been necessary had an appropriate dual diagnosis treatment program been in effect.

The project team developed a cause-and-effect analysis using the data from literature and the organization's activities, which included four major branches—limited services, inexperienced staff, lack of centralized processes, and loss of revenue—leading to limited dual diagnosis treatment (see Figure 2–5, page 50).

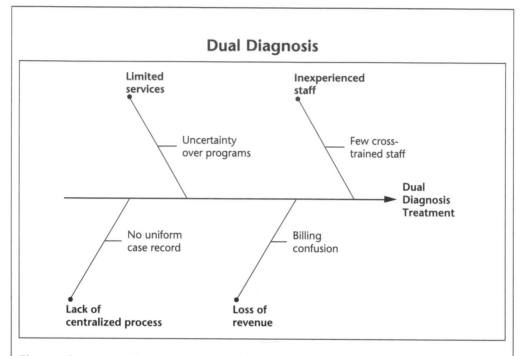

Figure 2–5 ■ *This cause-and-effect diagram illustrates a number of possible causes of system problems in dual diagnosis treatment.*

With the cause-and-effect diagram as a backdrop, the team entered a brainstorming, alternative solutions thinking, and planning phase. Out of this work came a number of clear mandates to

- adopt and articulate a philosophy of care,
- develop a method for insurance-triggered billing,
- identify cross-trained specialists in the health system,
- develop a unified screening device to identify dual diagnosis clients,
- establish regular meetings between mental health and chemical dependency staff,
- establish an initial level of dual diagnosis treatment by inter-departmental training programs,

- coordinate mental health and chemical dependency consultants as needed within 24 hours, and
- build and coordinate a comprehensive client tracking system to follow the client and gauge outcomes.

Results

The outcomes of this dual diagnosis project team included a number of positive results. An immediate improvement in staff morale was experienced as important treatment issues were being addressed throughout the health system. Immediately a new dual diagnosis treatment group was established, resulting in better utilization of appropriate levels of care and simultaneous gains in revenue and overall units of service. The dual diagnosis clients also experienced immediate improved clinical outcomes, since even the simple functions of triage and identification of these clients were facilitated by the new system. Finally, a more effective relationship between mental health and chemical dependency services and individual providers was established.

▣ Chapter Summary

Why Do We Design?

Design requires setting objectives based on

- the organization's mission, vision, and plans;
- the needs and expectations of the individuals served, staff, and others;
- current knowledge about organization and clinical activities;
- relevant data about performance and outcomes, and
- availability of resources.

What Do We Design?

■ Design focuses on functions and processes.

How Do We Design?

■ Successful designs are created by using a systematic method, basing decisions on data, involving the right people, and finding the best information.

Who Creates the Design?

■ Leaders set priorities for design.

■ The process' owners, suppliers, and customers create the design with other expert individuals as necessary.

3

Measure

"All science is measurement."

—Hermann Ludwig Ferdinand von Helmholtz

Measurement is essential to improve the quality of behavioral health care. It helps focus improvement efforts and provides tools to judge the effectiveness of treatments. In addition, public reporting of health care systems' performance measurements has taken on new importance in the health care marketplace.

No matter what process or function is examined (such as, group psychotherapy outcomes, psychiatric symptom changes, fire and safety education, orientation and training of residential care counselors, discharge planning, equipment maintenance, timely and comprehensive mental consultations) measurement can provide data that objectively describes how a function or process is operating and what its outputs are.

Measurement is by no means unfamiliar in health care. Many behavioral health care organizations routinely measure response to therapy, service length of stay, utilization of services, delivery response times, client satisfaction, equipment safety, staffing levels, and costs. This chapter discusses an overall rationale for measurement and how measurement works within the cycle for improving performance.

Recall the nine dimensions of performance (page 9). All are appropriate to consider for measurement.

In today's environment, accountability is an especially pressing concern. Behavioral health care organizations must demonstrate consistently and empirically that their care meets performance standards and must measure care outcomes, client satisfaction, and resource use.

To help behavioral health care organizations collect the data they need to improve performance, this chapter answers fundamental questions about measurement. This information will guide organizations in achieving one important result of measurement: a performance database that can be used to track performance, establish baseline data, and judge outcomes. Figure 3–1, page 55, highlights measurement's place in the cycle for improving performance.

For more detailed treatment of this subject, readers should consult two other Joint Commission books: *The Measurement Mandate** and *A Primer on Indicator Development and Application.*†

---

* Joint Commission on Accreditation of Healthcare Organizations: *The Measurement Mandate: On the Road to Performance Improvement in Health Care.* Oakbrook Terrace, IL: Joint Commission, 1993.

† Joint Commission on Accreditation of Healthcare Organizations: *Primer on Indicator Development and Application.* Oakbrook Terrace, IL: Joint Commission, 1990.

Cycle for Improving Performance—Measure

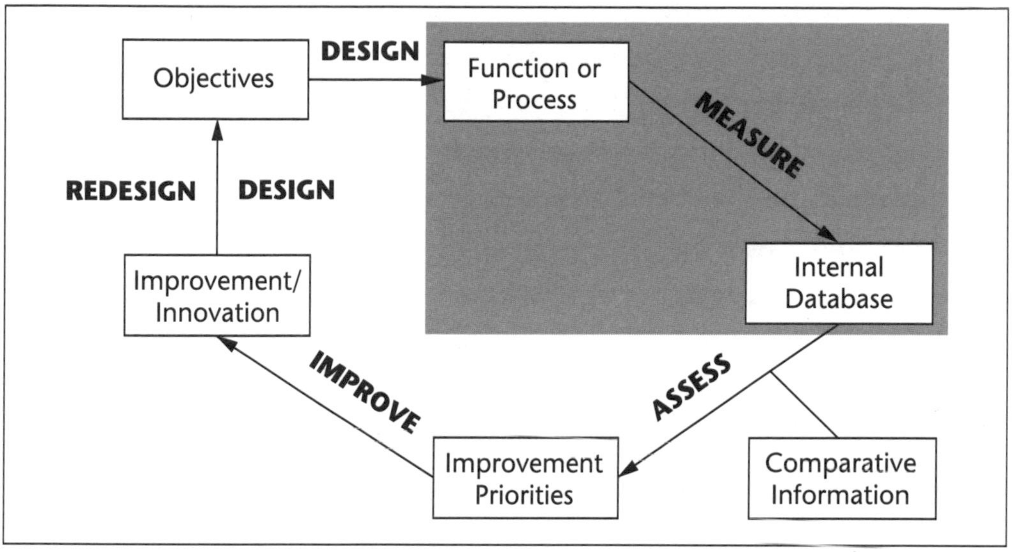

Figure 3–1 ■ *This figure highlights the **measure** stage of the improvement cycle—the subject of this chapter.*

▣ Why Do We Measure?

Chapter 2 described how to design a function or process. As new processes and functions are developed or existing processes are redesigned, a behavioral health care organization should collect data about its performance. Measurement is the process of collecting and aggregating these data, which help assess the level of performance. Measurement also determines if improvement actions are necessary. Finally, measurement provides evidence as to whether improvement has occurred.

One purpose of measurement is to provide baseline data. This is particularly important when little objective information exists about a process. For example, an organization may want to learn more about the current level of staff competence within a program, or staff may want to know more about the effectiveness of a new mental health service that supports individuals with psychiatric problems in their own homes and helps them avoid hospitalization or other institutionalization.

Specific indicators can be defined for a particular outcome or a particular step in a process, and used for ongoing performance assessment and improvement. Once assessed, these data can help staff determine whether a process is effective. Data about costs and benefits, including costs of faulty or ineffective processes, may also be of significant interest to organization leaders and can be a vital part of ongoing performance measurement.

Another purpose of measurement is to gain more information about a process chosen for assessment and improvement. For example, a target performance rate has not been met (such as a drug complication rate [too high] or a client/consumer satisfaction indicator [too low]); a performance rate varies significantly from the previous year, from work shift to work shift, or from the statistical average (for example, the average amount of time it takes to respond to requests for drug and alcohol screening significantly increases); or perhaps client or staff feedback indicates dissatisfaction with performance (for example, use of "time-out" procedures on an adolescent inpatient unit). Such findings may cause a behavioral health care organization to focus on a given process to determine opportunities for improvement. Detailed measurement would then be necessary to gather additional data about exactly how the process performs and about factors affecting that performance.

Finally, measurement helps to determine the effectiveness of improvement actions. For example, a behavioral health care organization that institutes a new process for early evaluation for a community residence program will not only need to establish a baseline rate for the existing process, but will need to continue measuring that rate after adopting the new process. Measurement can also be used to demonstrate that key processes (for example, the preparation, delivery, and administration of medications, or conducting and evaluating psychosocial group work) are "in control." Understanding variation over time and if a process is in fact in control (that is, within acceptable limits, with acceptable variation), is vital for continuous process improvement. Once a process has been stabilized at an acceptable level of performance, measures may be taken periodically to verify that the improvement has been sustained.

One very important end result of measurement is an organization-specific performance database. Such databases are invaluable for organization improvement and may contain linked information with reference points at multiple levels (for example, practitioner, program, and organization) about process performance, outcomes, satisfaction, cost, and judgments about quality and value.

Thus, measurement provides many benefits to organizations interested in continuously improving their performance. Several important benefits include the following (adapted from *The Measurement Mandate*):

- *Measurement creates a common language* that provides a degree of precision and clarity often needed to identify, analyze, and resolve important behavioral health care issues.

- *Measurement establishes benchmarks,* or points of reference, for performance. Benchmarks are used by organizations to identify potential opportunities for improvement and to determine performance improvement and degree of improvement. Benchmarks are increasingly being used by behavioral health care organizations, users, and payers of services to determine if their expectations for performance have been met.

- *Measurement provides organizations with data* that can be used to set performance improvement priorities.

- *Measurement improves the accuracy* with which behavioral health professionals observe, record, and form conclusions through data analysis about important processes and functions.

- *Measurement keeps health professionals clearly focused* on real improvement opportunities.

- *Measurement fosters participants' acceptance of, and involvement in,* the goals and processes of performance improvement activities.

- *Measurement provides milestones* toward which people can strive.

▣ What Do We Measure? Setting Priorities

An organization cannot and should not measure everything simultaneously. Its activities are too diverse and its resources too limited. Therefore, the organization's leaders, in concert with its staff, must find the most productive way to measure a wide range of the most important processes. One method is to measure certain outcomes or aspects of a process that can potentially identify larger performance issues. Determining what to measure is also related to what a behavioral health care organization defines as its work and prime deliverables. For example, a behavioral health care organization could measure the number of unexpected rehospitalizations of clients in a partial hospitalization program; a developmental disabilities clinic could measure its families' understanding of treatment procedures. When performance rates in important areas show significant variation or do not achieve targets, more detailed measurement and assessment should be initiated.

Leaders need to determine which processes will be subject to ongoing measurement. They must carefully weigh the processes' relationships to the organization's mission, vision, and resources. In addition, the concerns, needs, and preferences of the provider, the individuals served and their family, the community, purchasers, physicians, referral sources, and payers must be considered.

Table 3–1, page 59, depicts one possible method of identifying important processes to measure, assess, and improve. Using this methodology, an organization may periodically survey its clients, physicians, employees, and payers to help identify priorities for process measurement and improvement. For example, a drug and alcohol treatment facility may highlight potential processes to evaluate by developing a crosswalk of an assessment of customer perspective, listing key themes in the drug and alcohol standards, identifying the organization's important therapeutic and work processes, and reviewing the Joint Commission's nine dimensions of performance.

Table 3–1 ■ Example Methodology of Identifying Important Processes to Measure, Assess, and Improve

Customer Perspective	Key Drug and Alcohol Standards	Key Therapeutic and Work Processes	Performance
Client and families	Biopsychosocial assessments	Individual psychotherapy	Efficacy
Staff and management	Cognitive assessment	Group interventions	Appropriateness
Organization and governance	Neuropsychiatric functioning	Medication administration and effectiveness	Availability
			Timeliness
Community and key affiliations	Spirituality	Family work	Effectiveness
	History of dependency		Continuity
External evaluators HMOs, insurance			Safety
	Basic medical care		Efficiency
			Respect and caring

Other important factors to consider when choosing processes to continuously measure include standards or requirements from regulating or accrediting bodies, including the Joint Commission. For example, the Joint Commission identifies a number of important functions that may be the subject of ongoing measurement. This list of functions is worth considering because it provides a frame of reference for a behavioral health care organization conceptualizing its measurement activities. Measurement activities can also be organized around client diagnosis, critical paths, product and service lines, and other factors. These functions are broad and the associated standards intentionally allow considerable flexibility for measurement within each function.

For behavioral health care organizations, the standards address the following important functions.

Individual-focused Functions

- Rights, responsibilities, and ethics;
- Continuum of care, including the pre-entry and entry phases, care provided within the organization, and the pre-exit and exit phases;
- Assessment;
- Care, including treatment planning, anesthesia care, medication use, nutritional care, rehabilitation care and services, special treatment procedures, and treatment in forensic services; and
- Education, including individual and family education and responsibilities, and academic education.

Organization Functions

- Improving organization performance;
- Leadership;
- Management of the environment of care;
- Management of human resources;
- Management of information; and
- Surveillance, prevention, and control of infection.

Within these functions, specific processes or outcomes may be selected for measurement. The processes or outcomes typically chosen will

- affect a large percentage of clients;
- place individuals at serious risk if not performed well, performed when not indicated, or not performed when indicated;
- have been or are likely to be associated with problems;
- are costly; or
- represent cross-organization functions (for example, integrative processes).

The standards also identify certain important sources of data for measuring performance that a behavioral health care organization should consider, including

- Staff, individuals served, and others' views about the organization's performance, perceived problems, and opportunities for improvement;
- Risk management activities; and
- Quality control activities, especially in clinical laboratory services.

Customer Satisfaction and Experience

Individuals and their families are the ultimate focus of health care. Therefore, behavioral health care organizations should measure client satisfaction and experience with all aspects of care. Crosswalking client experience with the nine dimensions of performance, and integrating this information with organization-wide efforts will improve traditional components of patient satisfaction:

- Personal aspects of care,
- Technical quality of care,
- Accessibility and availability of care,
- Continuity of care,
- Convenience to the individual served,
- Physical setting,
- Financial considerations, and
- Efficacy of treatment.

Feedback from individuals served, families, physicians, referral sources, and staff can help an organization determine what process needs attention or identify a process' weaknesses and strengths.

▣ Who Performs the Measurement?

The staff responsible for performing measurement activities will differ depending on the goals and nature of the measurement undertaken. Two important ideas helpful in conducting measurement activities are: 1) tailoring and superimposing these activities into existing, ongoing data collection activities and 2) timing these activities as close to the occurrence of the measurement events as possible. The following sections provide some general guidelines on who may be responsible and involved in designing and collecting data for measurement.

Staff Involved in Ongoing Measurement to Monitor a Process

Some organizations are fortunate to have various experts who can help to design measurement activities, including experts in information management, quality improvement, and the specific functions to be measured. Other organizations without in-house expertise need to form strategic alliances with other groups or import these talents from elsewhere. At a minimum, the organization's leaders must review and approve the design of measurement activities.

Information management professionals and those responsible for carrying out the process being measured are key players in data collection. The people involved vary widely depending on the specific organization, on the process being measured, and on the measurement process. As noted earlier, organizations should make every effort to coordinate ongoing measurement with data collection already taking place as part of everyday activities. In addition, organizations should develop comprehensive data dictionaries that define the data elements, recording cycles, and owners of the processes.

Staff Involved in Measurement for a Specific Improvement Effort

This type of measurement is typically more detailed than routine screening. When an organization has decided to improve a particular process (for example, adverse drug reaction reporting, client education about medication side effects), it can empower a specific group to study the process, and recommend and implement changes. This group could be an existing team or a special team composed of those involved in the process studied. This team is usually responsible for designing and carrying out the measurement activities necessary to determine how the process performs. After making changes to improve the process, the team should continue to apply some or all of its measures to determine if the change has had the desired effect.

▣ How Do We Measure? Types of Measurement

Behavioral health organizations carry out several basic types of measurement:

- Ongoing measurement of selected outcomes or aspects of the process that most powerfully influence the outcome;
- Measurement of priority issues chosen for improvement; and
- Measures collected for one purpose that can be used to examine another process or function (secondary analysis approach).

The first type of measurement is related to quality control activities. The second method is part of more intensive assessment and improvement efforts, which may be initiated based on the results of ongoing measurement and performance data. The third is a practical method to collect important data without generating a new data-gathering effort. The measurement and analysis of any data may provide insight into multiple processes.

For example, a behavioral health care organization may continuously collect data regarding the number of completed referrals to a crisis care outpatient behavioral health team from the emergency room within 24 hours of referral. If that rate shows excessive variability or unacceptable performance levels, further assessment concerning the care referral and intake screening process should be initiated. This entails a more frequent, detailed data collection that addresses what type of clients are at greatest risk for hospitalization, a lack of caregiver support or an unsafe physical environment in the home, inadequate discharge preparation from the emergency department before linkage to the outpatient team, or the lack of adequate medications or supplies in the home. If an improvement is subsequently made in the intake screening or hospital emergency department discharge-teaching process, outcomes should be tracked closely to determine the effect of the change.

▣ Indicators

An indicator is a valid and reliable quantitative process measure or outcomes measure related to one or more dimensions of performance (such as effectiveness or appropriateness). The characteristics of an indicator and its components are shown in Table 3–2, page 65, and are more fully defined in the following paragraphs.

Key indicator characteristics include the following:

- *Quantitative.* Quantitative data represent information expressed in specific measurement units. These data do not, alone, express any judgment or conclusion about the process being measured. They provide specific, objective information requiring further study, analysis, and interpretation.

- *Valid and reliable.* An indicator is considered valid if the measurement correctly captures the event of interest, identifies an opportunity for improving performance, or identifies a phenomenon that merits further review, which is a step toward identifying an improvement opportunity. An indicator is considered reliable if it yields the same estimate by the same observer on multiple occasions or when it yields the same estimate by multiple observers of the same event. Reliability estimates confirm that you have obtained the same measurement for the same event consistently.

Indicators typically identify either a specific element of the process being measured or an outcome of that process. Outcomes measurement is necessary to learn results from improvement efforts and may record existing levels of and changes in health status, knowledge or behavior relevant to future health status, and satisfaction and experience with care personnel. Process measurement is designed to identify what caused those results.

In any behavioral health care organization, the relationship between process and outcomes is complex. Hence, outcomes do not directly assess quality of performance, but they permit an inference about the process of

Table 3-2 ■ Indicator Defined

An indicator is

> **Quantitative**—expressed in units of measurement
>
> **Valid**—identifies events that merit review
>
> **Reliable**—accurately and completely identifies occurrences
>
> **A measure of process**—a goal-directed series of activities
> **or outcome**—the results of performance

care. Also, because the outcomes of many clinical processes may not be evident or measurable at the time of specific events (for example, discharge) or may vary considerably due to patient-specific factors, it is prudent to measure the processes that most profoundly influence the anticipated outcome and the outcome itself.

An example of an outcomes indicator is "individuals with a diagnosis of a depressive disorder who demonstrate reduced depressive symptomatology and increased function." A process indicator might be "During formal clinical evaluation, individuals with a diagnosis of a depressive disorder receive an assessment for the potential to harm themselves or others." An outcomes indicator for environmental and life safety services might be "the number of staff who can correctly perform a fire drill procedure upon request."

Types of Indicators

Two types of indicators are sentinel-event indicators and aggregate-data indicators. A sentinel-event indicator identifies an individual event or occurrence that is significant and defined to trigger further review, study, and investigation each time it occurs. Most sentinel events are highly undesirable and occur infrequently. The following are several examples of sentinel events in a behavioral health setting:

- A completed suicide,
- Situations requiring seclusion and physical restraint of a client,

- A client who does not return from a day-pass,
- A client complaint of negligent staff, or
- A discharge against clinical advice.

Such indicators are well known in risk management. In quality management systems, they help ensure that each adverse event is promptly evaluated to prevent future occurrences.

Although sentinel-event indicators are useful to help ensure some basic functions (for example, client safety), they are less useful in measuring the overall level of performance in an organization. This is particularly true when they are the only indicators of organization performance because of the rare occurrence of these events, and because they often represent special as opposed to common-cause variation in organizations. A specific-cause or special-cause variation represents a unique set of circumstances not regularly present in the system. To mount a quality improvement effort based on special-cause variation, as if it were common, by introducing a fundamental change to the system would be a mistake.

An aggregate-data indicator, in contrast, quantifies a process or outcome related to many causes. Unlike sentinel events, an event identified by an aggregate-data indicator may occur frequently. Aggregate-data indicators are divided into two groups: rate-based indicators and continuous-variable indicators.

Rate-based indicators. Rate-based indicators express information in proportions. Typically, the proportion of the number of occurrences to the entire group within which the occurrence could take place are shown, as in the following examples:

$$\frac{\text{individuals with depression who develop suicidal ideation}}{\text{all individuals with depression}}$$

$$\frac{\text{child and adolescent psychiatric clients who are restrained/secluded}}{\text{all child and adolescent psychiatric clients with behavioral problems}}$$

$$\frac{\text{drug and alcohol clients who are HIV positive}}{\text{all drug and alcohol clients}}$$

The rate can also express a ratio comparing the occurrences identified with a different, but related, phenomenon. For example,

$$\frac{\text{individuals with depressive symptoms}}{\text{total outpatient visits for depression}}$$

Continuous-variable indicators. This type of aggregate-data indicator measures performance along a continuous scale. For example, a continuous-variable indicator might track the number of appropriate and "on task" behaviors per day for a schizophrenic client or the number of appropriate activities of daily living for a developmentally disabled client. Or it might record the number of visits and the time required for a behavioral change (for example, decrease in impulsive actions). Where as a rate-based indicator might express the proportion of the delivery responses that are greater than two hours to the total delivery responses, a continuous-variable indicator would measure the specific delivery response time, thus offering more precise information.

Those designing measurement activities must consider the process being measured, the goals of measurement, and the available data to choose the best type or types of indicators. Table 3–3, page 68, summarizes the different types of indicators; the examples in this chapter provide illustration of how indicators are used to measure performance.

Using Indicators

When selecting or developing a measurement system, staff should consider several important concepts to ensure balance. First, consider different types of measures to illuminate various aspects of the process (for example, measures of process and outcome, sentinel-event and aggregate-data indicators). Second, for each process or function being measured, the appropriate dimensions of performance should be considered and indicators should be tailored to address them. No single dimension eclipses the others; all are essential for an organization pursuing excellence in performance.

Figure 3–2, page 69, illustrates the interrelationships among important functions, client populations (for example, clients receiving specified

Table 3–3 ■ Types of Indicators

Aggregate data indicator: A performance measure based on collection and aggregation of data about many events or phenomena. The events or phenomena may be desirable or undesirable, and the data may be reported as a continuous variable or as a discrete variable (or rate).

> **Continuous variable indicator:** An aggregate data indicator in which the value of each measurement can fall anywhere along a continuous scale (for example, the number of visits in an outpatient clinic or the number of days between psychiatric hospitalization).
>
> **Rate-based (or discrete variable) indicator:** An aggregate data indicator in which the value of each measurement is expressed as a proportion or as a ratio. In a proportion, the numerator is expressed as a subset of the denominator (for example, clients who need dual diagnosis services versus all active patients). In a ratio, the numerator and denominator measure different phenomena (for example, the number of clients with depressive symptoms versus the number of disability days attributable to depression).

Sentinel event indicator: A performance measure that identifies an individual event or phenomenon that always triggers further analysis and investigation; it usually occurs infrequently and is undesirable in nature (for example, client adverse incidents).

---

services such as behavioral health care or chemical dependency treatment), and dimensions of performance. Any of these factors may provide the impetus for measurement and serve as a gateway to performance improvement. After determining what measures will be most useful, an organization could examine the linkages between the client population, dimensions of performance, and important functions. For example, a behavioral health care provider measuring care provided to developmentally disabled clients might focus on appropriateness or efficacy (dimensions of performance) of behavioral training (an important function).

The Quality Cube

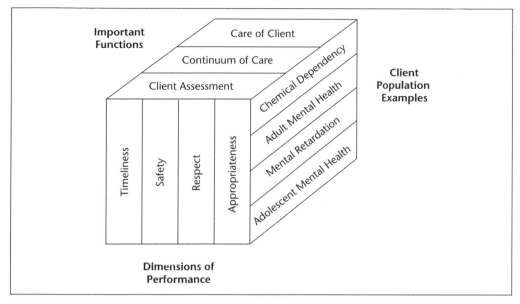

Figure 3–2 ■ *This figure illustrates the interrelationships among some dimensions of performance, some important functions, and some client population types.*

Examples of Measurement

◉ **Example 3-1: Quality Assessment: Measurement and Improvement in Psychotherapy Groups**

Note: This measurement effort, in the context of a larger, more comprehensive monitoring and evaluation program, proved to be a practical, positive, and cost-effective method for assessing and improving the quality of group psychotherapy in a clinical setting. As part of its improvement effort, a project development team created two new useful assessments focused on group psychotherapy services. These indicators became an important part of an ongoing evaluation and improvement process within the psychiatric services area. The example also provides a useful, easy-to-use, streamlined approach to assessing group psychotherapy practice in clinical settings and assessment of group leaders' competency skills.

Opportunity

A psychiatric service, part of a medical center, was interested in developing a methodology for monitoring, evaluating, and improving its group psychotherapy practice. In essence, this project team wanted to develop a monitoring program that would provide quality assessments, educational tools for quality improvement, and feedback to therapists.

The group psychotherapy practice for this particular medical center was a high volume service and was considered an important therapeutic factor in the overall service delivery system; hence its relevance as a clinical area for assessment. Their first challenge was to develop simple tools that would provide reliable and valid assessments of their ongoing group psychotherapy practice. A project improvement team was formed with multi-disciplinary team members. One of their first steps was to conduct a literature review in search of existing assessment tools. A review of a variety of available resources and additional other materials yielded no suitable empirical indicators focused on group psycho-therapy practice.

Assessment Approach and Implementation

The project team began its work with an overall survey of activities within the psychiatry area to determine the number, location, orientation, and leadership characteristics of existing psychotherapy groups. Early in the work the team met collectively with the psychotherapy group leaders to explain the intent and procedures associated with a monitoring program, emphasizing the educational and quality improvement goals of the program. This was a vital part of the effort and ensured a collaborative working environment within the service area.

Next, the team focused on development of two key indicators to assess group psychotherapy "process"—an *external indicator,* which essentially examined if group psychotherapy was clearly prescribed within a unit's treatment program and integrated into the overall treatment planning; and an *internal indicator* to examine if the group psychotherapy sessions were conducted within professionally accepted clinical guidelines. The external indicator, which involved the integration of group psychotherapy into the treatment planning process, included 1) unit has a written policy and procedure for patient participation in group psychotherapy, 2) unit policies implemented, and 3) group psychotherapies documented as part of the treatment plan.

Perhaps more relevant for the assessment of quality of group psychotherapy itself and demonstrated competence in group psycho-therapy, the internal indicator included such items as 1) therapist listens to and hears each group member, 2) therapist gives feedback to group members about their behavior, and 3) therapist is sensitive to group members' levels of participation. Additional items were also used with an educational goal: 1) therapist attends to non-verbal cues, and 2) therapist works in-depth with group members' feelings. It is important to note that these indicators are fairly straightforward, can be documented easily, and yield empirical profiles of group psychotherapy practice.

After developing the indicators, the team began pilot testing, and soliciting feedback and suggestions from the psycho-therapy group leaders and administrative and clinical managers. The team then conducted two 6-month periods of observation, data collection, and analysis. In addition, they conducted an inter-rater reliability study for pairs of raters across each indicator and clusters of individual items.

Outcomes

A number of positive outcomes emerged from this quality improvement effort including the following:

- Overall, the effort of monitoring group psychotherapy was generally viewed as a success in relation to improving quality assessment and developing an improvement measure.

- A detailed report of findings, conclusions, and recommendations provided important information to the psychiatry service's quality assurance committee of efforts to improve and document improved care.

- Through the validity and reliability study, the measures demonstrated adequate psychometric properties, making them practical and useful for research and clinical assessment.

- A multidimensional assessment system, including two types of process measures (one focusing on the integration and documentation of group psychotherapy practices into the treatment plan and the second focusing on the actual group leadership and group psychotherapy skills of the group leaders) was created. The second indicator also has important implications for demonstrating current competency.

- A positive response to the indicator development and monitoring system, particularly with regard to its educational and training features, was documented by feedback from individual clinicians, administrators, and group leaders.

- Estimated reductions in cost for quality improvement monitoring were realized over time.

▣ Example 3-2: Measurement of Treatment Planning in a Residential Children's Center

Source: Adopted from Price SB, Greenwood SK: Using treatment plans for quality assurance monitoring in a residential center. *Qual Rev Bull* 14:266–274, 1988. Reprinted with permission.

Note: This measuring and monitoring system enables administrators and staff to ensure treatment plans have been continually modified to take into account new information, new insights, and both improvements and setbacks. This measurement system with feedback allows the organization to empirically examine its performance in a vital clinical process.

Opportunity

This example describes how a residential children's center developed a plan for monitoring the form and content of treatment plans to satisfy the requirements of payers and accrediting organizations, and to contribute to the quality of care. The setting is a private, not-for-profit agency that provides a variety of short-term and long-term programs for mentally ill children and dysfunctional families. Approximately 150 children—mostly adolescents—receive residential treatment in campus-based cottages or community-based group homes.

Context and Setting

The center provides multidisciplinary services. Master's-level social workers provide case coordination and act as primary therapists, while psychiatrists' and psychologists' roles are to evaluate and consult with the social workers. Sociotherapists (child care workers) staff the living units and are responsible for supervising the children's routine activities, as well as intervening in crises. Nurses, under the guidance of a pediatrician, monitor the children's health care needs. Other rehabilitative services are provided by special education teachers, recreation therapists, art therapists, dance therapists, and others.

Length of client stay varies from six months to more than two years. Clients exhibit a wide variety of emotional and behavioral disturbances; the most common psychiatric diagnosis is conduct disorder, often complicated with borderline personality traits or borderline to mildly retarded intellectual functioning.

In general, the treatment goal is to reduce destructive behaviors and to help the children acquire interpersonal and self-care skills to resume living with their families, to live independently, or to success-fully continue treatment at a lower level of care (for example, group home or foster family home).

Treatment Planning Measurement

Within the center, treatment planning is viewed as an acquired skill that facilitates communication among service providers and gives direction to clients while requiring staff to analyze how best to use the available time and resources. Both the mechanics and the strategy are considered important components of a treatment plan.

The center mandates that the treatment plan's content, or strategy, should incorporate a realistic assessment of what can be accomplished with limited time and resources during the course of treatment. The service provider or consultant must develop realistic goals based on information obtained during the initial assessment of the child's history and emotional and intellectual status. In addition, the provider or consultant must envision the steps necessary to accomplish these goals.

The treatment plan's form must be complete and clearly presented in order to communicate the treatment strategy in a detailed and unequivocal manner. The rules referred to as the "mechanics" of treatment planning for organizing and presenting treatment plans are drawn largely from the requirements of the Joint Commission and other external accrediting agencies.

Some of the components of a treatment plan are outlined in Table 3–4, page 76. Several key elements of treatment plans are described in the following sections.

Initial assessments. Before the formal, comprehensive treat-ment plan is formulated, several assessments must be completed: health, psychiatric, psychological, social, behavioral, educational,

Table 3–4 ■ Components of a Comprehensive Treatment Plan

Initial assessments (completed before plan is developed)

Psychiatric diagnosis

Specific discharge planning

Level of client's participation in treatment plan development

Level of client's ongoing participation in the treatment process

Level of family's participation in treatment plan development

Level of family's ongoing participation in the treatment process

Strengths of the client and family

Client's major clinical needs or problems

Problem list updated as needed to include newly identified problems and to indicate when problems are reduced or resolved

Treatment goals

Service objectives

Service modalities for each objective

Rationale/justification for the plan

Date of next plan review (within 30 days for Medicaid-funded programs or 90 days for all other programs)

Signatures of case coordinator and supervisor, including dates

---

and recreational. These assessments include an overview of the client's status, test results and diagnoses, and recommendations for treatment.

Formulation of clinical needs and identification of strengths and weaknesses. As material from the client's history, evaluations, and interviews is gathered, the case coordinator begins to outline the client's strengths, weaknesses, and needs. This information is recorded in the "strengths" and "problem list" sections of the treatment plan.

Review of services available and admission justification. It is important to confirm that the current program and services are, in fact, the most appropriate for the client.

Establishment of the permanency goal. Identify the final destination of all children placed outside their homes (return to family, adoption, independent living, or adult residential services).

Timetable and treatment length expectations. What is a realistic estimated time available for this "treatment episode"? The treatment plan must reflect what can reasonably be achieved given each case's constraints.

Formulation of discharge criteria. The discharge criteria are the conditions that must be met before a client is ready to leave the program. Realistic and achievable discharge criteria presuppose a thoughtful application of all steps in treatment planning.

Therapeutic approach. The plan includes the relative mix of services and specific therapeutic modalities to be used. The coordinator must consider whether all the recommendations of the assessment providers can be implemented immediately or at any time during the treatment episode. For example, does the child need intensive individualized recreation therapy, or can he or she get adequate benefit from routine group activities? If school was the primary site of admission problems, should the plan emphasize behavior improvement in school rather than in the cottage?

Treatment goals. The first set of goals should clearly relate to the problems that pose the most serious impediments to further treatment; these goals usually focus on cessation of dangerous behaviors. The case coordinator should be able to visualize just how each goal will be achieved and should avoid inappropriate goals.

Objectives. Written by the team members and consultants who perform the assessments, objectives are the milestones on the way to achieving a treatment goal. They reflect the desired effect of treatment on the client, not the actions of the service provider.

Modalities. Each objective must be associated with one or more treatment modalities—the tasks and methods used by the service provider to help the client achieve the objective. Modalities, too, must be realistic.

Concurrent Review of Treatment Plans

As part of this system, quality assurance (QA) staff reviewed all comprehensive treatment plans (including the relevant assessments) and all formal treatment plan reviews after they have been written by the case coordinator and approved by the clinical supervisor. If there are mechanical problems (for example, missing signatures, obsolete target dates, or incomprehensible objectives), the plan is returned to either the case coordinator or the supervisor for immediate correction. If there are problems with the treatment strategy, the plan is returned to give the case coordinator an opportunity to clarify the plan before it is referred for a second-level review. If there are no apparent problems, the plan is filed in the case record.

The elements of the concurrent review process are outlined below and include the following:

- Structural details of the plan, including
  —clinical importance (for example, presence of measurable goals and objectives),
  —technical requirements (for example, dates, signatures),
  —teamwork (for example, presence of reviews by all providers in case), and
  —timeliness of plan review and documentation.

- Level of compliance with criteria expected for each case.
- QA staff action if criteria not met.
- Aggregation (quarterly summaries by case coordinator and assessment provider to providers, supervisors, program directors).
- Standards (level below which action plan is required): 75% for treatment plan appropriateness (no more than one in four plans returned for mechanical problems); 14-day average for plan documentation turnaround; 90% for clinical assessments appropriateness.

Treatment plan mechanics are reviewed to ensure that each element is complete, timely, and comprehensible. Because the treatment plans have now achieved a high degree of mechanical quality, more emphasis is being placed on the strategic aspects.

A typical plan review takes from 8 to 35 minutes. Because QA staff are also responsible for training service providers to perform QA activities, they occasionally spend additional time with service providers who have trouble conceptualizing goals and objectives.

Strategic problems are also reviewed and related to either the quality or the appropriateness of care. Problems relating to the appropriateness of care are referred for discussion and recommendations. Quality problems are referred to program-specific quality assurance review committees and include assessment of the following:

- *Appropriateness.* A treatment plan is inappropriate if either the program as a whole or specific service components are not appropriate for a particular child.
- *Criteria for length of stay.* Admission criteria for continued stay is another common measure of program appropriateness. Although a wide variation is expected, outliers can be identified and should be examined closely.

■ *Quality.* Monitoring the quality of care through treatment plans is the organization's most difficult—but perhaps its most important—undertaking. Quality problems may also raise the question of staff competence. Typical issues may include the following:

—Changes from what originally was thought to be a realistic discharge plan (for example, can the client return to the community or family life) to a less ambitious destination should be examined.

—Failure to achieve objectives over time not only may lead to a review of the program's appropriateness for the client, but also may call into question the provider's competence to formulate achievable objectives and effective service modalities.

—Was the objective too ambitious for the time allowed? (For example, a child reduced his runaway incidents by 25%, but not by the expected 50%.)

—Was the objective off track because the provider expected behavior that the client simply was not ready to exhibit or skills that the client had not yet acquired?

—Was the modality not intense enough; that is, sessions that were too infrequent or too short? (For example, a client is responding well to a life skills group and appears to understand the material at the end of each session; however, he forgets everything between the sessions, which are conducted every two weeks.)

The purpose of periodic and systematic review of objectives and modalities is to ascertain what is working and what is not.

Another important aspect of quality of care is how the service providers and the treatment system react to crises. Critical events include episodes with important implications for the client's life and future treatment, including the following examples:

- A child makes a serious suicide attempt;
- An adolescent becomes pregnant;
- A child commits a crime and is sent to jail or detention; or
- Staff discovers that a client has been engaging in prostitution or intravenous drug use.

Patterns of less serious occurrences (for example, increase in restraints or runaway episodes) and distinct changes in symptoms or problem patterns are also important to review carefully to ascertain the treatment response.

Timely and aggressive discharge planning is also critical to a successful discharge and to ensure a smooth transition back to family or to another treatment program.

Results

Treatment plan monitoring and measurement with feedback has had several effects:

- Staff take treatment plans very seriously; consistently poor performance is eventually reflected in performance evaluations.
- Identification of lapses in treatment and of strategic thinking and monitoring have resulted in well-organized treatment plans.
- The organization successfully satisfies a wide range of external surveyors.
- The review system is also the cornerstone of the agency's QA plan—one that efficiently blends a multitude of disciplines and helps the agency avoid establishing monitoring systems for each one.

> ■ Most importantly, this system, in conjunction with the agency's other monitoring systems, encourages the organization to be a self-questioning and self-renewing organization.

▣ Chapter Summary

Why Do We Measure?
- To gain information about performance on an ongoing basis;
- To gain detailed information about a process chosen for assessment and improvement;
- To determine the effects of improvement actions; and
- To produce organization-specific performance databases.

What Do We Measure?
- Selected high-volume, high-risk, problem-prone, or costly processes on an ongoing basis;
- Selected processes, as indicated by ongoing measurement or other feedback;
- Customer experience and satisfaction; and
- Cross-functional, cross-discipline processes.

Who Performs the Measurement?
- Leaders with input from many sources (for example, staff, consumers, governance) decide what to measure on an ongoing basis;
- Organization experts can help design ongoing measurement activities;
- Information management professionals and those responsible for a process are key players in data collection; and

- Work groups or other teams measure processes chosen for intensive assessment and improvement.

Indicators

- An indicator is a valid and reliable quantitative measure related to one or more dimensions of performance;
- Indicators can identify sentinel events or can show aggregate performance;
- Two types of aggregate-data indicators are rate-based and continuous-variable indicators; and
- Indicators can measure processes and outcome.

One Product of Measurement Is a Performance Database

- The database provides aggregate information about process performance, outcomes, satisfaction, cost, and judgments about quality.

▣ References

Hamilton JD, et al: Quality assessment and improvement in group psychotherapy. *Am J Psychiatry* 150(2):316–320, 1993.

Nadzam DM, et al: Data-driven performance improvement in health care: The Joint Commission's Indicator Measurement System (IMSystem). *Jt Comm J Qual Improv* 19(11):492–500, 1993.

Price SB, Greenwood SK: Using treatment plans for quality assurance monitoring in a residential center. *Qual Rev Bull* 14:266–274, 1988.

4

Assess

"'I urged them to work with the vendors and to work on instrumentation.' I said, 'You don't need to receive the junk that comes in. You can never produce quality with that stuff. But with process controls that your engineers are learning about—consumer research, redesign of products—you can. Don't just make it and try to sell it. Redesign it and then again bring the process under control... with quality ever-increasing.'"

—W. Edwards Deming in *The Deming Management Method*

- Why Do We Assess?
- What Do We Assess?
- Who Performs the Assessment?
- Assessment Techniques
- Assessment Tools
- Examples of Assessment
- Chapter Summary
- References

Once data are collected as part of measurement, they must be translated into information and used. Behavioral health care organizations can use such information to make judgments and draw conclusions about performance. This assessment forms the basis for actions taken to improve performance. Assessment activities include identifying the root causes of problems, determining the current performance, and interpreting any variations in process or outcomes that suggest that improvement may be necessary.

Figure 4–1, page 87, illustrates assessment's role in the improvement cycle. One vital function of assessment is the use of comparative information and internal organization data to set improvement priorities. This may include benchmarking activities as well.

▣ Why Do We Assess?

Assessment activities answer these questions:

- What are the problems that need to be solved?
- What processes or functions can we improve?
- What are the priorities among these opportunities for improvement?

Assessment is particularly important when a new process is developed. When a behavioral health care organization designs a new process, it should measure its performance and compare the resulting data to design specifications and customer expectations to determine if the process is performing well.

When an organization measures an existing process, it should assess whether the process is stable, what its capabilities are, and whether its outcomes are consistent with expectations.

As a new process is designed or an existing process is redesigned, we are most interested in a variety of process measurement, including

- process stability,
- process capability, and
- process outcome.

After variation has been determined, assessment of data can identify the size and the types of variation and point out potential opportunities for

Cycle for Improving Performance—Assess

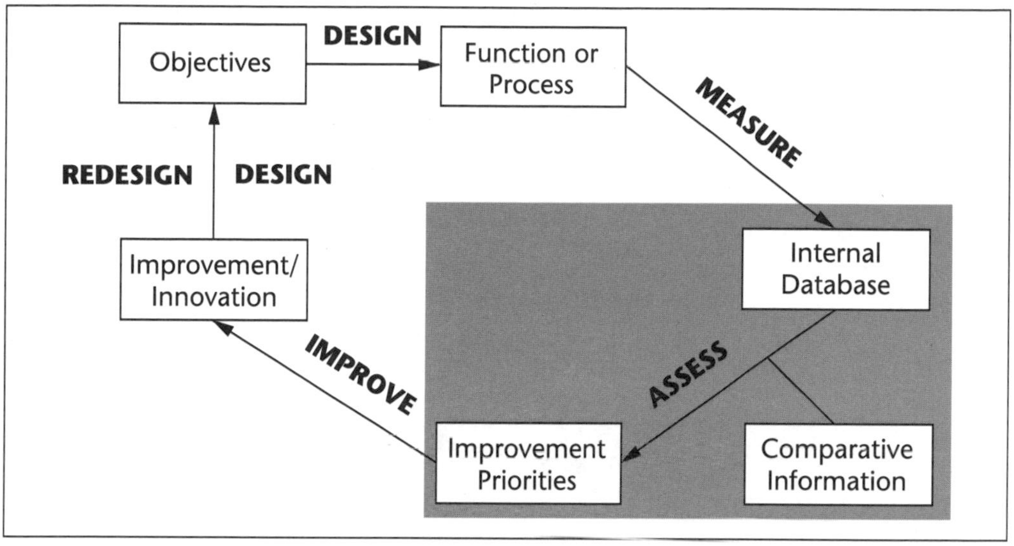

Figure 4–1 ■ *This figure highlights the **assessment** stage of the cycle for improving performance. It includes the comparative information this activity requires and the improvement priorities that result.*

improvement. Even if a process is stable, assessment might reveal additional opportunities for improvement. However, because of limited time and resources, organizations will not be able to take action to address all opportunities for improvement and, therefore, must set improvement priorities among existing identified opportunities.

Once an organization determines that an improvement effort is warranted, it must identify the root causes behind that performance. These causes will be the prime targets for any improvement actions.

After an organization takes action to improve performance, it must continue to collect and assess data in order to determine whether improvement occurred; that is, whether undesirable variation was reduced or eliminated, or whether the capability of the process and associated outcomes were improved.

Assessment is not confined to information gathered within the walls of a single behavioral care organization or even a collection of facilities under a larger single health care system. To better understand its level of performance, an organization or system needs to compare its performance against reference databases, professional standards, trade association guidelines, and other sources. It is also important to recognize that these standards are also dynamic and ever changing, requiring a constant comparative process.

▣ What Do We Assess?

Assessment can be divided into two types: routine assessment, which uses data from ongoing measurement, and special assessment, which is part of focused improvement efforts.

Routine Assessment

Data from all ongoing measurement should be assessed. How often assessment occurs depends on the process being measured, the organization's priorities, and the nature and types of indicators. For example, a CMHC may assess client complaints immediately, whereas it may assess data pertaining to the process of new client orientation and education every quarter. A chemical dependency organization might review data about appropriate use of psychoeducational groups every two months and data about client and family satisfaction with overall services every six months. Similarly, a school-based treatment program for mentally retarded/developmentally disabled clients may assess the use of time-out daily, but review data about the client and family education on generalization of behavioral programs to home settings each week in the context of a treatment plan review. Routine assessment should always be reviewed from the standpoint of "How often to measure? How often to review?"

Special Assessment

At times, routine assessment will suggest that a more intensive study of a process is warranted. This could include more detailed measurement and assessment, more frequent data collection intervals, use of secondary analysis of other data relevant to the process, or more intensive analysis of the data available. More intensive assessment (or measurement and assessment) is typically triggered under the following conditions:

- By important single events, such as those identified by sentinel-event indicators (for example, a serious injury to a client, a significant treatment complication, an unexpected death);
- By a performance level that varies significantly from an absolute level established by the organization, sometimes called a "threshold for evaluation";
- By patterns or trends that significantly vary from those expected, based on appropriate statistical analysis (for example, initiating more intensive assessment when performance is two or more standard deviations below the mean);
- When the organization's performance significantly varies from that of other organizations or from recognized standards; and
- When the organization wishes to improve already acceptable performance levels.

The Joint Commission's standards state some outcomes should trigger more in-depth assessment, including

- significant life safety errors,
- all significant adverse drug reactions,
- significant errors related to medication use, and
- client rights violations.

Each state may also have a list of critical adverse events requiring reporting.

▣ Who Performs the Assessment?

Both routine and special assessments may be performed by a number of staff and consumers. Routine assessment is typically performed by those who designed the measurement method or by others with a solid knowledge of statistics, the process being measured, the reference points against which performance is compared, or the criteria for triggering more intensive special assessment.

Special assessment usually includes the people closest to the process being addressed: those who carry out or are affected by the process. Remember also the importance of cross-discipline/cross-service quality improvement efforts when considering who performs the assessment. Service, discipline, or office-location barriers cannot be allowed to limit participation in improvement efforts. When a process involves more than one service, the group improving the process should reflect all services. By including the process's participants, and sometimes consumers, the organization not only taps the necessary expertise, it also helps ensure the necessary understanding and support for the recommended changes.

▣ Assessment Techniques

The primary goals of assessment, as mentioned previously, are to determine where performance can be improved, to set priorities for improvement, and to evaluate the effectiveness of actions taken to improve performance. In general, this requires some review of the organization's performance outcome, comparisons with performance of other organizations, and possibly identification of local or national "best practices."

Comparing Data

Most types of assessment and assessment of performance require comparing data to some point of reference. The reference points may include

- historical patterns of performance in an organization and, if available, with internal longitudinal databases;
- aggregate external reference databases;
- practice guidelines/parameters and clinical pathways/protocols;
- desired performance targets, specifications, or thresholds; and
- expected outcomes.

Historical patterns of performance in the organization. When an organization has accumulated sufficient data, it will be able to compare current performance to its own historical patterns. This allows the organization, in effect, to act as "its own control group" and evaluate performance. For example, an organization might compare current performance levels with levels taken from the previous year. It could also compare performance levels for various days of the week, shifts, or parts of the organization. With good data over a significant period of time, an organization can develop its own standard error of measurement estimates and empirical guidelines to help define control limits for a given process.

Perhaps one of the most common and useful comparisons using historical data involves analyzing the variation in the process. Variation is inherent in every process; performance measured by indicators will never be static. Consider, for example, that an organization is measuring turnaround time for completion of psychosocial assessments. The turnaround time cannot be identical for each assessment conducted, but should conform to basic expectations. For another example, consider a managed care organization that is measuring the effect of a health promotion program (for example, weight management or smoking cessation) or a social support program for depression. Obviously, not all participants will show the same result. In other words, results will vary.

Distinguishing the type of variation present is important, because each type of variation will require a different type of action for improvement. Variation has two general types and causes. One is called *common-cause variation*. This is the random variation inherent in every process. For example, in a smoking cessation program each participant has a variety of personal factors that affect his or her ability to stop smoking: working conditions, family support, smoking history, and so forth. A process that varies only because of common causes is said to be *stable*. A stable process, one with only common cause variation, can be improved.

A second type of variation is called *special-cause variation.* This type arises from unusual circumstances or events that may be difficult to anticipate. These causes result in marked variation and an *unstable* process. Human error and mechanical malfunction are examples of special causes that result in variation. For example, in a weight management or smoking cessation program, a special cause of variation might be a counselor who misses a session or a participant and counselor who do not speak the same language. Special causes of variation must be systematically identified and eliminated; however, removing a special cause will only eliminate aberrant performance, not improve the basic level of performance. A much more fundamental improvement comes from studying the process and improving its design. Failure to distinguish the types of variation can lead to two types of errors: reacting to special-cause variation as if it were common and reacting to common-cause variation as if it were special. Both errors are common.

Aggregate external reference databases. In addition to assessing its own historical patterns of performance, an organization should compare its performance with that of other organizations. This kind of comparison will be increasingly important in the future when access to organization data across the country is facilitated through more advanced telecommunications. Expanding the scope of comparison helps an organization draw conclusions about its own performance and learn about different methods to design and carry out processes.

Aggregate external databases take various forms. Aggregate, risk-adjusted data about specific indicators produced by these databases can help each organization set priorities for improvement by showing whether its current performance falls within an expected range.

National multi-office systems also often have system-wide databases that feed back information about certain indicators (for example, client outcomes [such as satisfaction] or behavioral health care utilization data [such as the average number of visits by discipline category and client diagnosis]) to regional or branch offices for use in their individual performance improvement activities. Hospital-based behavioral health care that is part of a larger health system may initiate collection of similar data for comparison with other behavioral health care organizations. Several state and federal professional and trade associations have recently initiated comparative databases in which members may participate. Typically, payers also aggregate information about performance and cost, as do states and the federal government.

Practice guidelines/parameters. Practice guidelines/parameters, critical paths, and other standardized client care procedures are also very useful reference points for comparison. Whether developed by professional societies, in-house practitioners, or clusters of health care organizations, these procedures represent an expert consensus about the expected practices for a given diagnosis or treatment. Assessment variation from such established procedures can help an organization identify opportunities for improvement and build the foundation for research.

Desired performance targets. Organizations may also establish targets, specifications, or thresholds for evaluation against which they compare current performance. Such levels can be derived from professional literature or expert opinions within the organization. For example, based on the clinical literature, available depression research, and past organization performance, an organization may set the following as complementary targets:

- Primary care physicians who treat depressed patients should refer those patients to a mental health professional if they do not respond to treatment within 12 weeks; and
- 95% of all depressed patients recommended for a medication trial must receive an adequate trial of antidepressant medication as evidenced by appropriate therapeutic levels and time course.

Assessment and improvement activities should strive to help an organization create new processes or redesign existing ones to meet their desired performance targets.

Benchmarking

One method of comparing performance is benchmarking. Although a benchmark can be any point of comparison, most often it is a standard of excellence. Benchmarking is the process by which one organization studies the exemplary performance of a similar process in a similar organization and, to the greatest extent possible, adapts that information for its own use. Or the organization may wish to simply compare its results with those of other organizations or with current research or literature. For example, a behavioral health care organization wanting to further study its processes for employee recognition and retention might want to review local, state, or national trends on employee attrition in the workforce. Or a chemical dependency treatment program may want to compare its clients' relapse rates to those of other providers.

The organization may look to non-health care organizations to further examine processes used to enhance employee retention, such as training, promotion strategies, and employee recognition programs.

Studying the patterns of care or service in another organization often results in an infusion of new ideas—ideas that never would arise if the assessment and comparison remained within one's own walls. The organization serving as the benchmark or "best practices" model can benefit, as well. By discussing the process in question—by reexamining each step and its rationale—that organization may also gain new insights. Figure 4–2, page 95, illustrates one approach to successful benchmarking.

Assessing Factors That Affect Performance

More intensive assessment requires learning what factors cause the current performance and its relationship to outcomes. This is achieved by studying a process; learning its steps and critical decision points; identifying the various people, actions, and equipment required for the process's outcomes; finding links among variables in performance; and ranking the frequency of causes. Tools such as flowcharts, cause-and-effect diagrams, and Pareto charts—described later in this chapter—are useful in studying a process and identifying potential areas for improvement.

Four Steps to Benchmarking

Step 1	Step 2	Step 3	Step 4
Plan	Collect	Analyze	Adapt
• Decide what to benchmark	• Collect information on your own process	• Compare processes and identify gaps	• Set improvement goals
• Select team	• Identify benchmarking partners	• Identify characteristics of superior performance	• Close performance gaps
	• Collect information from partners	• Determine how to close the gap	

Figure 4–2 ■ *This figure illustrates one approach to benchmarking.*

Source: Adapted from Flower J: Benchmarking. Springboard or buzzword? *Healthc Forum J* 36(1):14–16, 1993. Reprinted with permission.

Setting Priorities for Improvement

Setting priorities for measurement and improvement is a critical step in any quality effort. Throughout the improvement cycle, organization leaders must set priorities for deciding what to measure, what to assess, and what to improve. Deciding what to improve is perhaps most important because of the significant investment of time and effort involved as well as the potential effect on organization-wide performance.

A behavioral health care organization's leaders play a key role in setting priorities for improvement. Leaders are often in the best position to view the organization's overall goals, the availability of resources to address the improvement opportunities, and the organization-wide effect of change in process and outcome. Priority-setting decisions reflect behavioral health care research, expert judgment, and information, combining epidemiology, diagnostic understanding, therapeutic efficacy, and anticipated cost/benefit of improvement. Leaders also need input from the appropriate people, departments, units, teams, and offices in the organization.

Priorities for improvement are dynamic and ever changing. They can be influenced in various ways, such as by

- a sentinel event that requires immediate improvement action;
- a new or modified strategic direction from the governing body or organization leadership;
- the initiation of a new service or service location;
- a change in the organization's structure, such as by a joint venture or acquisition;
- client/family feedback;
- recent clinical developments and innovations;
- referral source, physician, community, or payer feedback; and
- legislative and community health care reform actions.

An organized approach to setting the priorities for improvement should be as objective and comprehensive as possible. Organizations might consider creating a set of selection criteria to use in this process that indicates a range of organization priorities. The following list suggests possible selection criteria:

- *The degree to which the opportunity reflects the organization's mission, philosophy, goals, and policies.* If, for example, one of the organization's key strategic goals is to improve and expand its home-based behavioral health care services, a project to train volunteers and institute a community outreach program might be desirable.
- *Whether the resources required to pursue the improvement opportunity are available.* Some improvements—such as minor procedural changes— require relatively few resources; others require more substantial amounts of time (for example, creating a critical path, redesigning a clinical service) and funds (for example, establishing a new service, opening a new branch location). The resources required must be weighed against the resources available and the benefits expected. In

some cases, the lack of resources necessary to make an improvement will result in the opportunity being assigned a lower priority.

- *Whether the opportunity affects one of the client care and organization functions identified in Joint Commission standards.* The functions significantly affect the care clients receive and the organization's ability to provide that care.

- *Whether the improvement opportunity addresses a high-volume, high-risk, or problem-prone process.* For example, a high-volume process for many organizations is likely to be clinical assessment and education efforts. A high-risk process might be administering electroconvulsive treatment in an outpatient setting. A problem-prone activity might be arranging an out-of-home placement for a violent adolescent.

- *The degree to which the opportunity reflects clients' priorities with respect to their needs, preferences, and expectations.* In a behavioral health care organization, clients and their families or care givers are critical customers. It is essential to know what their needs and health care experience have been.

- *Whether the opportunity pertains to a high-impact clinical service.* Such services may include medication use; mental health and psychosocial care of HIV-positive clients; care of suicidal clients; and use of restraint and seclusion.

- *Whether the opportunity pertains to utilization management, risk management, and/or quality control concerns.* These areas are typically of high priority in behavioral health care organizations. For example, a quality control concern for an organization might be routine review of mental status post detoxification, or assessment of potential for violence in a partial hospitalization program.

- *Whether the opportunity addresses a high-cost function or process or whether the opportunity promises significant cost savings.* The pressing need to provide care efficiently makes potentially cost-saving changes high-priority opportunities. An example for any behavioral health care organization would be training and retaining qualified staff. By improving its processes for staff orientation and ongoing training, the organization might find that it is able to retain its experienced staff, thus saving the costs of frequently recruiting and orienting new staff. It might also improve staff ability to function in key areas (for example, life safety, client care functions).

■ *Whether the opportunity for improvement represents a cross-discipline, cross functional aspect of performance.* The emerging Joint Commission standards and experience in quality improvement efforts emphasize the importance of cross-discipline, cross-functional care delivery.

Assessing Individual Performance

Most widespread and fundamental improvement arises from attention to processes and systems. However, at times measurement and assessment will also identify individual performance as the cause of variation. In that case, intensive assessment, review, and recommendation, and any appropriate action and follow-up are required.

Each organization is expected to have detailed procedures for addressing a problem in an individual's performance (for example, individual counseling, education, responsibility changes, required consultation). The organization's leaders are responsible for assessing the competence of staff members.

Although individual performance issues will continue to arise, it is vital to remember these tenets of performance improvement:

■ The vast majority of behavioral health care professionals are skilled, knowledgeable, and dedicated.

■ The vast majority of improvement opportunities lie in processes, not individuals.

■ Some of the best opportunities for improvement lie in integrative work (for example, connections between different services for the same client over time) and core processes (essential functions).

▣ Assessment Tools

For continuous improvement of care, tools and methods are needed that document observations, build knowledge, and share understanding with others. This section provides a quick overview of a few tools and methods for performance assessment. These simple but powerful tools can be learned quickly and utilized effectively by all organization members.

Statistical Tools

Three statistical quality control tools are especially helpful in comparing performance with historical patterns and assessing variation and stability: run charts, control charts, and histograms.

Run charts. A run chart (also known as a time plot) plots points on a graph to show meaningful trends in levels of performance over time. It also can demonstrate trends, such as movement away from the average. It can help identify which existing processes need improvement and can show whether an action taken to improve performance was successful. Figure 4–3, below, plots

Run Chart

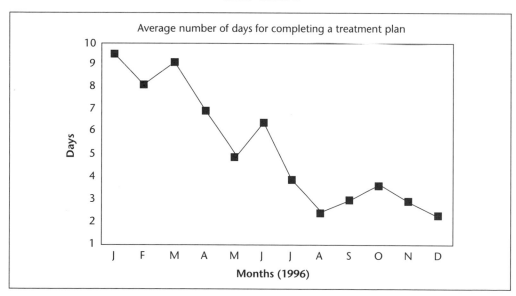

Figure 4–3 ■ *A run chart displays points on a graph to show levels of performance over time.*

the average turnaround time for completing the care plan for each month in 1996. Leaders with system knowledge can use run charts to track operating indicators.

Control charts. Adding computed limits (control limits) to a chart increases the value of a longitudinal record. A control chart is a run chart with the addition of a statistically derived upper control limit (UCL) and lower control limit (LCL). It shows variation in a process and helps discern whether that variation is due to special or common causes. When performance variation is random and stays within the UCL and LCL, the causes of the variation are considered common causes. When performance exceeds the upper or lower control limits, or demonstrates specific predictable patterns within the control limits, the variation is due to a special cause. Figure 4–4, below, shows an example of a control chart. It is

Control Chart

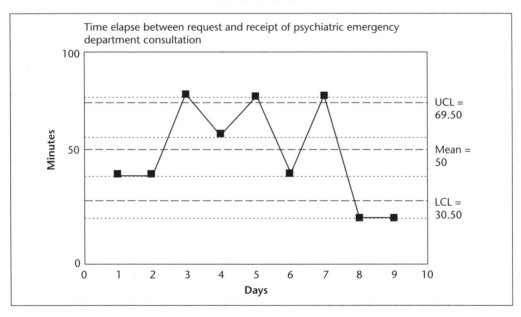

Figure 4–4 ■ *A control chart is a run chart with upper and lower control limits (UCLs and LCLs) added; they are usually two or three standard deviations from the mean. Their purpose is not to indicate whether the process is running at the desired level, but whether it is statistically in control. This example shows time elapsed in minutes between request and receipt of psychiatric emergency department consultation.*

important to note that control limits are not the same as specification limits, budgets, targets, goals, or objectives. They only indicate what the process is capable of, not what the process is expected to perform or what the process designers hope to achieve.

Histograms. Histograms show the pattern of variation in a process or its outcomes. For example, consider that the production time to produce a completed and signed psychosocial assessment after interview can range from one to five days. This variation may seem unpredictable, but it generally follows some pattern; therefore, the range of variation is predictable. In most cases, the variation is expected to fall within a normal distribution. For example, perhaps normal production time (for non-emergency situations) is expected to be between one and two days. This indicates that a referral source could call within two days and expect to receive information on the assessment most of the time. At times, however, the distribution is not normal and is unpredictable. This may signal the need for further evaluation. Histograms illustrate these ranges of variation. Figure 4–5, page 102, gives an example of a histogram along with instructions on creating one. The histogram is also related to the Pareto chart (refer to page 105).

Causal and Process Analysis

A number of tools are helpful for determining the root causes of current performance: flowcharts, cause-and-effect diagrams, scatter diagrams, and Pareto charts.

Flowcharts. Flowcharts are visual schematics that show step-by-step the unfolding of a process or a plan of an activity. A flowchart identifies the actual path that a process follows, as opposed to the one that may be defined in the policies and procedures manual. Flowcharts include top-down flowcharts, detailed flowcharts, workflow diagrams, and deployment charts. By documenting a process's sequence in steps in a flowchart, a team can identify redundancies, inefficiencies, misunderstandings, endless loops, waiting times, and inspection steps, which are the areas that create the biggest problems in most processes. This helps the team gain an understanding about

Histogram

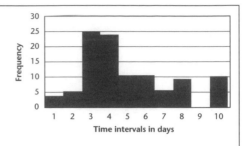

Use this procedure to create a histogram:

1. Obtain the data set and count the number of data points.
2. Determine the range for the entire data set by deducting the smallest value from the largest value.
3. Determine the number of classes (bars) into which the data set should be divided.
4. Determine the class width, which equals the range divided by the number of classes.
5. Determine the class boundaries.
6. Construct the histogram chart, placing the values for the classes on the horizontal axis and the frequency on the vertical axis.
7. Determine the number of data points included in each class and construct the bar graph.
8. Analyze the findings.

Figure 4–5 ■ *A histogram helps behavioral health care organizations discover patterns of variation in processes and outcomes.*

how the process should be performed. Once the actual process is illustrated in the flowchart, the team can create a flowchart to show the ideal path the process should take. It is safe to say that in many behavioral health care organizations, processes are being used that have never been described or fully studied, but have grown out of historical practice patterns.

Teams can use flowcharts at several crucial stages:

■ Designing new processes,

■ Designing a method for measuring a process,

■ Identifying problems,

■ Analyzing problems to determine causes, and

■ Planning solutions.

See Figure 4–6, page 103, for instructions on how to create a flowchart.

Flowchart

This procedure will help you create a flowchart:

1. Determine the starting and ending points of the process.
2. Brainstorm to record all the activities and decision points involved in the process. The brainstorming should be done by those people familiar with the various parts of the process.
3. Arrange activities and decision points in sequence.
4. Using this information, create a flowchart. Place each activity in a box and each decision point in a diamond. Connect them with lines and arrows to indicate the flow of the process.

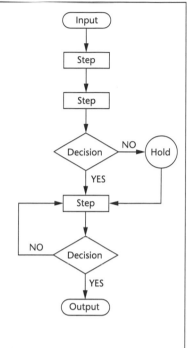

Figure 4–6 ■ *A flowchart illustrates the sequence of steps that a process follows.*

Cause-and-effect diagrams. A cause-and-effect diagram is sometimes called a "fishbone" diagram (because of its shape) or an Ishikawa diagram (after its creator, Kaoru Ishikawa). It enables the team to map out a list of factors thought to affect a problem or desired outcome. It can show a large number of possible causes of a particular outcome (including negative outcomes such as delays, medication errors, or client dissatisfaction). It is constructed using the experience and expertise of the process's customers and suppliers, and it shows how various components of the process relate to one another. Once completed, the diagram helps identify specific conditions requiring further attention and might suggest appropriate actions. In addition, a cause-and-effect diagram can provide ideas for data collection to measure performance. Cause-and-effect diagrams are considered most helpful to use when a process has been described and the problem has been well defined. An example of a cause-and-effect diagram is provided in Figure 4–7, page 104, along with a procedure for creating one.

Cause-and-Effect Diagram

To create a cause-and-effect diagram, follow this procedure:

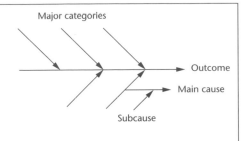

1. Place the outcome (or problem statement) on the right side of the paper, halfway down; draw a horizontal line across the paper with an arrow pointing to the outcome.
2. Determine general, major categories for the causes; connect them to the horizontal line with diagonal lines.
3. Note the main causes and place them under the general categories. The team will need a brainstorming session to determine the main causes.
4. List subcauses and place them under the main causes. To determine subcauses, ask *why* five times.

Figure 4–7 ■ *A cause-and-effect diagram depicts the large number of possible causes of a particular outcome.*

Scatter diagrams. Another useful assessment tool is the scatter diagram, which illustrates the statistical relationship between two variables. Groups use scatter diagrams when they want to examine a theory about the relationship between two variables, when they analyze raw data, and when they assess an action taken to improve performance.

In a scatter diagram, each variable is assigned an axis; points where the variables intersect are marked with dots. The shape of the scatter of points tells you if there is a relationship. If the points cluster in an area running from lower left to upper right, the variables have a positive correlation; if they cluster from upper left to lower right, they have a negative correlation. If there is no relationship, the points are scattered randomly over the graph. A scatter diagram may not conclusively prove a relationship, but it can offer some convincing evidence. Figure 4–8, page 105, gives more information on how these diagrams are created and includes a sample illustration.

Scatter Diagram

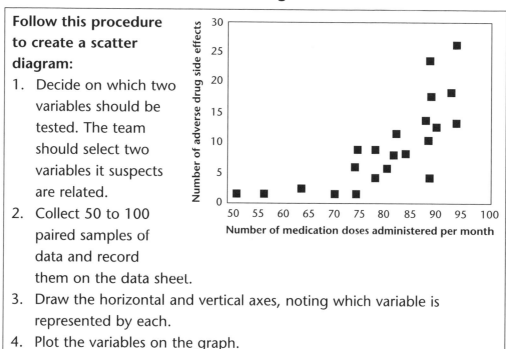

Follow this procedure to create a scatter diagram:

1. Decide on which two variables should be tested. The team should select two variables it suspects are related.
2. Collect 50 to 100 paired samples of data and record them on the data sheet.
3. Draw the horizontal and vertical axes, noting which variable is represented by each.
4. Plot the variables on the graph.

Figure 4–8 ■ *A scatter diagram illustrates the relationship between two variables.*

Pareto charts. A Pareto chart depicts, in descending order, the frequency of problems affecting the process being studied. This useful bar graph allows a group to categorize occurrences and focus on those that most frequently occur and are, therefore, most important. It is a natural follow-up to a cause-and-effect diagram. Having listed a number of causes, the group could use a Pareto chart to display their relative frequency. This information would, in turn, help a group decide which cause to address first. Figure 4–9, page 106, displays a simple procedure for how to put together a Pareto chart.

Decision Making and Planning

Two specific tools can be used to set priorities for improvement and help team decision making: selection grids and multivoting.

Pareto Chart

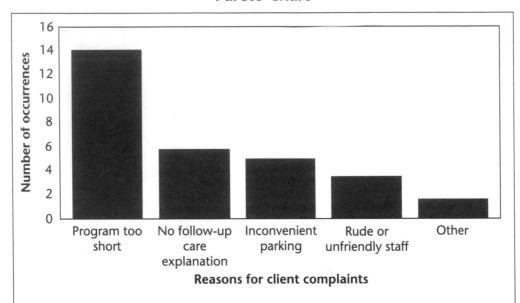

Use this procedure to create a Pareto chart:
1. Decide on the topic of study.
2. Select the type of causes or conditions to be compared. The team must choose the specific factors contributing to the outcome.
3. Determine the standard for comparison—this could be frequency, cost, or amount.
4. Collect data. Check sheets can be helpful for this step.
5. Compare frequency, cost, or amount (as appropriate) between categories.
6. Draw and label the vertical axis with the standard for comparison in increments.
7. Draw and label the horizontal axis with each factor in descending order.
8. Draw the bars to indicate the frequency (or cost or amount) of each factor.

Figure 4–9 ■ *A Pareto chart depicts in descending order (from left to right) the frequency of events being studied.*

Selection grids. A selection grid can be a useful tool for setting priorities for improvement. Figure 4–10, page 107, shows how this tool works. The horizontal axis of the matrix lists the selection criteria; the vertical axis lists

Selection Grid

Criteria / Issues	Quality of care	Client satisfaction	Staff morale	Cost	Total
Issue #1	X	X	—		x - 2 0 - 0 – - 1
Issue #2	0	X	X	—	x - 2 0 - 1 – - 1
Issue #3	—	X	0	X	x - 2 0 - 1 – - 1
Issue #4	—	—	X	0	x - 1 0 - 1 – - 2
Issue #5	0	—		—	x - 0 0 - 1 – - 2
Issue #6	0	0	—	X	x - 1 0 - 2 – - 1

Key to scoring

X = strong effect   — = weak effect
0 = some effect   = no effect

Figure 4–10 ■ *A selection grid helps set priorities for quality improvement. Each issue is examined for four criteria, with scores assigned for each. The answers can help a group see where its priorities actually lie.*

the improvement opportunities. Each person assigns a score to indicate the effect of a particular criterion on an opportunity. The points are totaled for each opportunity; higher totals suggest higher priorities. Responses to specific criteria may also help determine improvement priorities. For example, although the total was highest for issue #1, it may not be chosen as a focus for improvement if the group did not tend to agree that the issue affected the quality of client care.

Multivoting. Another tool for setting improvement opportunities is multivoting—a technique for narrowing a broad list of ideas to those that are most important. Each person involved in the multivote has a limited number of points to assign to a predetermined list of improvement opportunities. These can be given in any number to any of the possibilities, with the number indicating level of importance. Once the votes are tallied, the

Multivoting

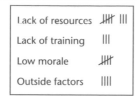

Lack of resources	JHT III
Lack of training	III
Low morale	JHT
Outside factors	IIII

Use this procedure for multivoting:

1. Using a predetermined list of ideas, consider whether any are duplicates or similar.
2. Ask the group—especially those who identified the items in question—whether similar items may be grouped together.
3. If the group agrees, combine the duplicate or similar items.
4. Number each item on the new list.
5. Determine the number of points that will be assigned to the list by each group member.
6. Allow several minutes for group members to independently assign their points to one or more of the items on the list.
7. Indicate each member's point allocation on the list.
8. Tally the votes for each item on the list.
9. Note the items that received the greatest number of points.
10. Choose the final group or multivote again.

Figure 4–11 ■ *Multivoting narrows a broad list of ideas to those that are most important.*

range of possibilities is usually narrowed to those the group considers most important. See Figure 4–11 above for a simple procedure for conducting multivoting.

Examples of Assessment

▣ Example 4-1: Quality Improvement Indicators for Outpatient Psychotherapy Opportunity

Note: This example highlights the use of detailed assessment of client and therapist perceptions of care and peer reviews of outcomes in psychotherapy. The two studies in this example describe investigated relationships among quality improvement indicators within a large outpatient behavioral health delivery system. The studies provide an example of the importance and use of process and outcomes assessments within outpatient behavioral health care and highlight the use of these ratings for quality improvement programs. They also foreshadow the important emerging value of clinical guidelines and standardized approaches to care, particularly with regard to therapeutic processes such as psychotherapy.

Introduction

An outpatient behavioral health care organization initiated a research-oriented quality improvement (QI) program focused on evaluating outpatient psychotherapy. This organization launched two studies examining the relationships among quality improvement indicators in psychotherapy practice, searching for common elements of effective treatment and trying to develop simple and cost-effective measures of treatment outcomes. The plan was designed from a QI perspective to eventually integrate an ongoing program of psychotherapy research into the development and tracking of QI standards, guidelines, and overall quality indicators. It was also thought that studying relationships among these indicators could be useful in a variety of ways. The assessments and indicators were undertaken in a large outpatient behavioral health care delivery system.

Two studies were initiated. The first examined the relationship between clients' and therapists' perceptions of treatment. A second study examined the relationship between clients' satisfaction with treatment and therapists' overall compliance with standards and practice guidelines.

Clients' and Therapists' Ratings

In the first study, clients completed questionnaires at the end of their treatment that measured satisfaction with their therapists' overall treatment and degree of perceived problem resolution. In a similar manner, therapists assessed their clients' improvement with two measures: a global assessment of functioning (which was rated at the beginning and end of treatment) and the same scale that the clients used to rate overall degree of problem resolution at the close of treatment.

Analysis of client measures indicated that clients were highly satisfied with treatment and overall ratings of problem resolution were moderately high (32% rated themselves as much or very improved and 63% reported moderate improvement). Therapist-rated functioning scores for clients also showed significant positive changes as a result of treatment. Additionally, therapists' ratings of problem resolution reflected a moderate degree of improvement, somewhat comparable to that judged by clients.

As expected, there were positive correlations between several outcomes measures, including clients' rating of satisfaction with a therapist and treatment ratings of problem resolution. Also, clients' ratings of satisfaction with the therapists correlated with the ratings of the overall satisfaction for the program. There was also significant concordance between the ratings of problem resolution by clients and therapists.

Assessment of Theory, Process, and Outcomes

The second study focused on therapists' compliance with standards of care and guidelines and clients' overall satisfaction with treatment. Foundation's Health PsychCare service developed these standards through a professional committee and distributed them to care providers as guidelines for assessment and treatment approaches, confidentiality protocols, and documentation requirements. The guidelines also included a variety of procedures to be used in monitoring therapists' overall compliance. Prior to implementation, therapists were involved in a series of training seminars when these guidelines were distributed.

Using the standardized guidelines, a panel made up of a variety of experienced service providers created a peer review format to review cases. The general protocol consisted of reviewing therapists' reports and associated clinical documentation (presenting problem, diagnosis, treatment goals, therapist strategy, and therapeutic strategy). The peer reviewers evaluated each case on completeness of material, consistency of diagnosis with assessment data, and consistency of therapy with diagnosis. After reviewing numerous treatment elements, each reviewer assigned a quantitative rating representing compliance with standards and guidelines. These ratings were then compared and correlated to clients' satisfaction scores.

Overall analysis indicated a relatively good degree of agreement among the peer reviewers' ratings of cases and client ratings. Not surprisingly, therapists were rated highly by peer reviewers and clients in almost all peer review components of treatment. In the process, some key problem areas were also found, however; these included inconsistency between assessment data and resulting diagnosis and lack of objective, attainable treatment goals.

Outcomes

From an assessment perspective, the ratings of therapeutic change and treatment satisfaction used in the studies were simple, cost-effective measures helpful for assessing treatment in a behavioral health delivery system. Data emerging from the peer review process is also useful and suggests some additional findings, namely, the value of identifying and establishing standards and guidelines, and the importance of including such guidelines in peer review processes. The findings with regard to comparisons between clients and therapists were also noteworthy. There was a relatively strong relationship between clients' ratings of satisfaction and peer reviewers' rating of therapist com-pliance. This may suggest that clients were more satisfied with short-term psychotherapy when their therapists were able to establish a good working relationship and follow a highly structured, goal-directed process. The results also suggest that 1) overall clients were satisfied with the treatment they received; 2) therapists and clients perceive moderate improvement as a result of treatment; and 3) clients' satisfaction was directly related to degree of perceived improvement.

From a quality assurance (QA)/QI perspective, satisfaction and the peer review ratings can be viewed as useful QI indicators yielding opportunities for both aggregate QA information and more individualized peer review competency profiling.

▣ Example 4-2: Assessment of Patient Satisfaction with Mental Health Services: A Meta-analysis to Establish Norms

---

Note: This example provides a method to estimate levels of patient satisfaction with various types of mental health programs and an approach toward using existing health services research for benchmarking purposes. Equally important, the example demonstrates the feasibility of developing such norms for assessment purposes and foreshadows the value of an accumulative database that could be updated on a regular basis. The example also emphasizes the importance of selecting measurement techniques that are specific to the type, and nature of patient characteristics under review.

Introduction

A program established in conjunction with a residency training contract between a state hospital and local university sought to assess the program's level of patient satisfaction as part of its overall quality assessment program. The unit was developed to assess and treat chronic young adult patients at the state hospital. Care emphasis was placed on reevaluation of their diagnoses and functional status, review of their treatment histories, prescription of well-monitored trials of various pharmacologic treatment, and provision of structured rehabilitation programs to improve their opportunities for community living.

Many of the patients admitted to the unit struggled with assaultive behavior, chronic suicidal tendencies, and significant noncompliance, and they were unresponsive to treatment. An ultimate goal of the program was to achieve community placement for patients who were considered "not placeable."

In concert with ongoing assessment of typical outcome variables, including discharge to community, length of stay, and frequency of problematic behavior, the clinical team also considered the issue of patient satisfaction.

Opportunity

A number of field trials were run to establish the validity and reliability of satisfaction measures, although the team became aware that many of the existing measures had no clear reference points. One option for developing such reference points was to consider pooling data from several studies, perhaps using meta-analytic techniques, to achieve an adequate comparison basis. It was thought that such comparisons would complement earlier evaluations and allow possible benchmarks and standards to emerge.

Plan and Analysis

To examine this problem, the team analyzed available literature. The first step was to develop a classification scheme for mental health programs along three critical dimensions: 1) inpatient compared to outpatient compared to residential care; 2) a chronicity of illness classification; and 3) conventional programs compared to new treatments. This classification scheme was critical to allow comparisons between types of care and also formed the basis to conduct a literature analysis of patient satisfaction according to program type. Perhaps of critical importance in this example is the team's use of an existing database in research literature as an opportunity to conduct an assessment within the team's own clinical program. Applying descriptive and statistical techniques to the available literature, the team explored a number of questions including 1) Does patient's satisfaction vary according to type of mental health program?, 2) What are the typical levels of patient satisfaction across all program categories?, and 3) Can preliminary norms of satisfaction be established for the various program types that have reasonably well-behaved distributions?

Findings

A distribution of satisfaction scores by program type indicated that the rates of satisfaction were exceedingly high (more than 50% for many of the programs). The distribution also indicated that a significant number of programs clustered around the average satisfaction level within confidence intervals for this distribution. In the future, analyses such as these will become increasingly important for benchmarking purposes and assessment comparisons outside local programs.

Additionally, the findings of overall positive levels of patient satisfaction also continue to highlight the need for specific program data against which to compare future evaluations, as well as more specific inquiry further tailored to the type and nature of health care delivered. Using additional equations and confidence intervals, administrators from other CMHCs or inpatient facilities could compare their assessments with the norms established in this program to gauge whether their individual findings would compare favorably with the existing literature.

▣ Chapter Summary

Why Do We Assess?

- To compare performance with various reference points;
- To determine root causes for current performance;

- To set improvement priorities; and
- To determine the effect of improvement actions.

What Do We Assess?

- Organization performance and care outcomes;
- Initial assessment of ongoing measurement; and
- Intensive assessment triggered
  —by important single events,
  —by certain performance levels and/or patterns or trends,
  —when the organization's performance varies significantly from that of other organizations,
  —when the organization's performance varies significantly from recognized standards, and
  —when the organization wishes to improve already acceptable performance.

Who Performs the Assessment?

- Groups that include the process's owners, customers, and suppliers, with additional expert input as needed.

Assessment Techniques

- Comparing performance with important reference points, including patterns of performance, external databases, practice guidelines/parameters, and desired performance specifications or thresholds.
- Identifying best practices.

Assessment Tools

- Run charts, control charts, histograms, flowcharts, cause-and-effect diagrams, scatter diagrams, Pareto charts, selection grids, and multivoting.

▣ References

Camp RC: *Benchmarking: The Search for Industry Best Practices That Lead To Superior Performance*. Milwaukee: American Society for Quality Control (ASQC) Quality Press, pp 16–21, 1989.

Flower J: Springboard or buzzword? *Healthc Forum J* 36(1):14–16, 1993.

Hargrave GE, Hiatt D: An analysis of outpatient psychotherapy: quality improvement indicators. *Managed Care Quarterly* 3(1):72–75, 1995.

Lehman AF, Zastowny TR: Patient satisfaction with mental health services: a meta-analysis to establish norms. *Eval Program Plann* 6:265–274, 1983.

Using Quality Improvement Tools in a Health Care Setting. Oakbrook Terrace, IL: Joint Commission, 1992.

Zastowny TR, Stratmann WC, Adams EH, Fox MI: Patient satisfaction and experience with health services and quality of care. *Quality Management in Health Care* 3(3):50–61, 1995.

5

Improve

"Toto, I've a feeling we're not in Kansas anymore!"

—Dorothy in *The Wizard of Oz*

- What Are the Goals of Improvement?
- Who Takes Improvement Actions?
- How Do We Improve Processes? Tools and Methods for Improvement and Innovation
- Examples of Improvement
- Chapter Summary
- References

Behavioral health care organizations are rapidly realizing that the world of health care has dramatically changed. Today organizations must be able to compete "anytime, anyplace, on anything" to survive and prosper.

The fundamental outcome of the framework for improving performance is improvement. Taken together, design, measurement, and assessment culminate in specific actions to improve performance. Improvements come about through redesign of existing processes or through innovation and design of new processes. Figure 5–1, page 120, shows the relationship of this phase to the rest of the cycle for improving performance.

Cycle for Improving Performance—Improve

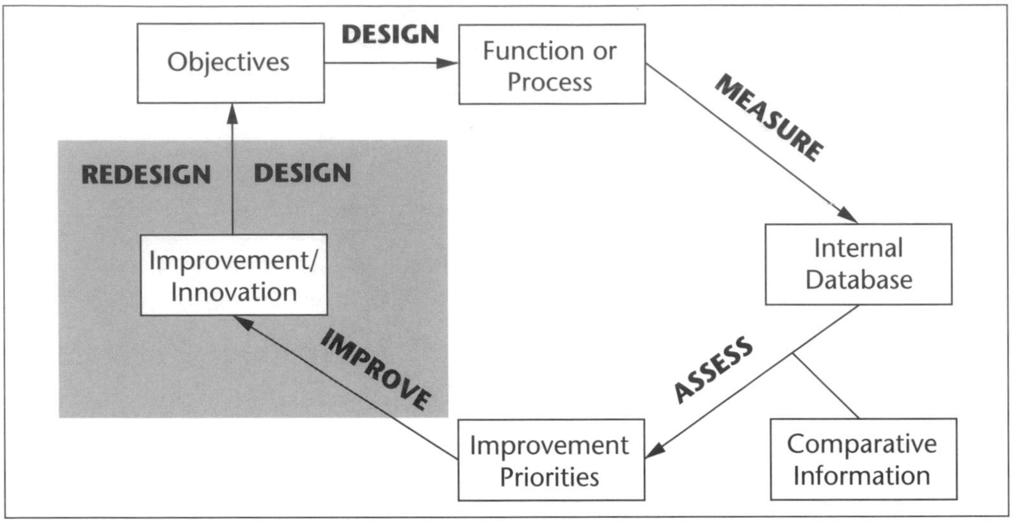

Figure 5–1 ■ *By adding* **improve** *and* **redesign/design**, *the cycle is complete.*

▣ What Are the Goals of Improvement?

Improvement is a continuous, never-ending process. Organizations should strive to continuously improve important functions. The following questions will help behavioral health care organizations set goals and develop a comprehensive plan for their improvement efforts.

What dimension(s) of performance will be most affected by the change? To understand the potential effects of the improvement activity, the organization must determine which dimension of performance (efficacy, appropriateness, availability, timeliness, effectiveness, continuity, safety, efficiency, and respect and caring) will be affected. At times, the relationship between two or more dimensions must be considered. For example, when a service's availability is increased, the process' efficiency may decline, but cost per unit of service may decrease. In Chapter 2, the design chapter, this understanding of goals for improvement will also be affected by the type and nature of the care delivered. For example, how does care delivered in a residential drug and alcohol program differ from treatment delivered in an inpatient psychiatric unit or a school for developmentally delayed children?

How are the dimensions of performance organized in each care environment?

How do we expect, want, and need the improved process to perform? The behavioral health care organization and the team carrying out the effort should set specific expectations for performance resulting from the design or improvement (for example, turnaround time for treatment plan updates will decrease by 20%). These expectations can be derived from staff expertise, patient/public expectations, experiences of other organizations, recognized standards, and other sources. Without these performance expectations, the organization will not be able to determine the degree of success of the efforts or judge its improvements overall.

How will we measure to determine if the process is actually performing at the level we expect? The organization and team will need specific tools to measure the performance of the newly designed or improved process in order to determine whether performance expectations are met. These measures can be taken directly or adapted from other sources, or they can be newly created, as appropriate. As always, the measurement will be subject to the traditional guidelines of the scientific method (for example, valid and reliable).

Who is closest to this process and therefore should "own" a portion of the improvement activity? To a great extent, the success of an improvement effort hinges on involving the right people from all disciplines, services, and offices involved in the process being addressed. For example, a discharge planning project from a halfway house might involve appropriate representatives from nursing, psychology, social work, case management, and administration, as well as physicians and clients. A life safety project in an adolescent residence might include clinicians, nursing staff, the clinical manager of the residence, a life safety expert, and the residents.

Processes and Individuals

Improvement actions should be directed primarily at processes. As stated earlier in this book, process improvement holds the greatest opportunity for significant change, whereas changes related to an individual's performance may have limited effect. In behavioral health care, as in other endeavors, good people often find themselves carrying out bad processes.

Individual performance cannot, however, be ignored. In behavioral health care, the possible consequences of skill, knowledge, or judgment problems are grave, sometimes life threatening. Therefore, when measurement and assessment direct attention to an individual's performance, appropriate action must be taken. This action often takes the form of counseling, education, or activity restriction. In the occasional cases in which care professionals will not or cannot address performance problems, other actions are necessary in accordance with policies and procedures, such as modifying their job assignments or scope of responsibilities. Behavioral health care organizations should consult the leadership and management of human resources standards in the most current copy of the *MHM* for more information on individual performance, assessment, and management.

▣ Who Takes Improvement Actions?

As with other phases of the improvement cycle, involving the right people from the beginning is essential. The process for taking action consists of several stages, each of which may have different players and teams.

Designing the Action

In general, the group that has measured and assessed the process should have the necessary expertise to recommend improvements and is in the best position to design the improvements. This group should include those who carry out or are affected by the process. The group may also import special expertise as needed in the design or evaluation process.

Approving Recommended Actions

When substantial resources are involved and the potential effects are significant, the organization's leaders will usually become involved in reviewing and approving the action. In other cases, a solution may be relatively simple to implement (for example, shifting duties within a service area, or changing a minor aspect of an existing process). Such a change usually can be approved by the appropriate manager. It is important to remember that if a group has obtained the necessary input and buy-in while devising an improvement, the final approval should come readily.

Testing the Action

Testing should occur under "real world" conditions, involving staff who will actually be carrying out the process under day-to-day operations. Effects can be measured with the same methods used to establish a performance baseline.

Implementing the Action

After careful piloting, full-scale implementation of a process change should have significant and positive results. However, any change can create anxiety. Therefore, care should be taken to prepare staff and clients for change and to explain the reason for the change in an educational, non-threatening way. Cooperation is viewed as essential for changes to succeed, and typically will not occur if people believe a change is being forced on them. An effective team should have already acquired much of the necessary buy-in during earlier phases of the improvement process. Appendix B, page 167, provides further suggestions for promoting effective teamwork in implementing improvement initiatives and highlights a model of progress for a project team.

▣ How Do We Improve Processes? Tools and Methods for Improvement and Innovation

Once the goals and priorities for improvement have been established, the organization can begin planning and carrying out innovations. A standard, yet flexible, process for carrying out these changes should help leaders and others to ensure that actions address root causes, involve appropriate people, result in desired and sustained changes, and ultimately improve outcomes. The fundamental components of any improvement process include:

- Defining the problem/opportunity for change,
- Testing the change,
- Studying its effects, and
- Implementing changes determined to be worthwhile.

The Scientific Method

Many readers will readily associate the activities listed above with the basic scientific method. Indeed, the scientific method is the fundamental, inclusive paradigm for change, and includes these steps:

1. Determine what we know now (about a process, problem, topic of interest).
2. Decide what we want to learn, change, or improve.
3. Develop a hypothesis about how the change can be accomplished.
4. Test the hypothesis.
5. Assess the effect of the test; compare results "before versus after" or "traditional versus innovative."
6. Implement successful improvements or re-hypothesize and conduct another experiment.
7. Generalize the innovation to all relevant areas.

This orderly, logical, inclusive process for improvement will serve behavioral health care organizations well as they assess *and improve performance.*

Plan-Do-Check-Act

A well-established process for improvement that is based on the scientific method is the plan-do-check-act (PDCA) cycle. This process is attributed to Walter Shewhart, a quality improvement pioneer. It is also widely associated with W. Edwards Deming, a student and later a colleague of Shewhart. Deming made the PDCA cycle central to his influential teachings about quality. The cycle is compelling in its logic and simplicity. A brief explanation of this process should help readers not already familiar with PDCA to understand and use the cycle (see Figure 5–2, page 126).

Plan. During this step, an operational plan for testing the chosen improvement action is created. Small-scale testing is necessary to determine whether the improvement actions are viable, whether they will have the desired result, and whether any refinements are necessary before putting them into full operation. The list of proposed improvement actions should be narrowed to a number that can be reasonably tested.

During the planning stage, several issues should be resolved:

- Why is the idea being tested?
- Who will be involved in the test?
- What do they need to know to participate in the test?
- What are the testing time tables?
- How will the test be implemented?
- What are the success factors?
- How will the process and outcomes of the test be measured and assessed?

Do. This step involves implementing the pilot test and collecting actual performance data.

Check. The data collected during the pilot test are analyzed to determine whether the improvement action was successful in achieving the desired outcome(s). To determine the degree of success, actual test performance is compared to desired performance targets and baseline results achieved using the established process.

Act. The next step is to take action. If the pilot test is not successful, the cycle repeats. Once actions have been shown to be successful, they are made part of the standard operating procedure.

These are the key steps of the PDCA cycle.

- Plan:
    —Determine data needed to monitor the improvement in the process.
    —Determine tests for the improvement monitoring plan.

PDCA Cycle

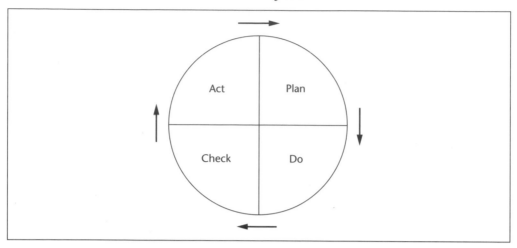

Figure 5–2 ■ *The PDCA cycle is useful in planning, testing, assessing, and implementing an action to improve a process.*

- Do:
  —Collect and analyze data on improvement in the process.
  —Make improvement changes/actions when indicated and appropriate.
- Check:
  —Establish decision/review points to determine the effectiveness of changes.
  —Assess the effects of improvements.
  —Analyze the improvement results.
- Act:
  —Meet on a regular basis to determine what was learned.
  —Repeat tests or actions, if necessary, to ensure improvement in the process.
  —Generalize improvements.

The process does not stop here. The effectiveness of the action should be continually measured and assessed to ensure that improvement is maintained.

Tools for Making Improvements

Many tools used for measurement and assessment are also useful for taking action to improve processes and enhance team decision making:

- Brainstorming can be used to create ideas for improvement actions.

- Multivoting and selection grids can help a group decide among various possible improvement actions.

- Flowcharts can help a group design a new process or redesign an existing one.

- Cause-and-effect diagrams can describe causal flow and indicate possible causes that an action should address.

- Pareto charts can show the effects of improvement actions on root causes.

- Run charts and control charts can measure the effects of a process change.

- Histograms can show changes in variation as the result of an action.

See the assessment tools text, page 99, for more information.

Critical Paths

One significant improvement method not yet discussed is the critical path (also referred to as the clinical path, clinical or critical pathway, and practice guideline).* Several factors have converged to spur the development of critical paths, including 1) ongoing cost containment forces, 2) total quality management initiatives to reduce practice variation, and 3) emergence of consistent and reliable treatment approaches. Critical paths offer a

---

* While these terms are often used interchangeably, there are some differences. The terms are all included under a definition of "practice protocols"; *critical pathways* are a treatment regime, with consensus of clinicians that include only a few elements proven to affect patient outcomes; *clinical pathways* are similar, but broader and include all elements of care; *practice parameters* represent an agreed upon strategy for patient management deemed acceptable practice by professional organizations. (*Hosp Risk Manage* 16(2):20, 1994).

systematic, flexible guide for client care. They include descriptions of acceptable methods to diagnose, manage, treat, or prevent specific diseases and conditions.

Such guides can be used by psychiatrists, psychologists, nurses, social workers, therapists, addiction specialists, and other staff to guide—but not mandate—the care delivery process. They are designed by those involved in the process—clients, psychiatrists, psychologists, nurses, social workers, therapists, and others—who come together to offer their unique perspectives and expertise. It is important to note that the guideline path must be seen as a continuous cycle, incorporating ongoing development and outcomes assessment with updating and revision.

A critical path is an excellent way to approach the design of the process for a new service or a complete redesign for an existing process that needs change. One advantage of a critical path is the opportunity to start fresh, cast aside traditional but not particularly effective procedures, and research and implement the best practices.

Selecting the process. The initial step in creating a critical path is choosing a process to standardize. If an organization is planning to launch a new service, the process for path design may be self-evident, but is less so when an organization wants to redesign an existing process. Behavioral health organizations perform a wide range of diagnoses and procedures, treat a variety of conditions, and offer services at a variety of levels of care. Likely candidates for redesign are processes that are high volume, high risk, problem prone, costly, important to staff or patients, key to the organization's mission, or represent a cross-discipline, cross-functional process.

Defining the boundaries of the path. The critical path can begin anytime during the episode of care and can also stop at any time. For example, critical paths can start well before admission. One integrated hospital-to-home-care critical path might follow the client across settings and continue after discharge.

Defining the diagnosis, condition, or procedure. An appropriately defined process and client population to be served will simplify critical path development. Identify as clearly and precisely as possible the client population for whom the path is designed. A process that is too broadly defined will result in a path that is either too complex or too vague; conversely, a process that is too narrowly defined can result in a path that applies in only a limited number of cases. For example, a behavioral health care agency may begin its critical path development by defining the most frequent patient diagnoses served in the previous year and studying approaches to assessment and treatment in this group (for example, all individuals with a first depression episode).

Forming a path design team. The group that creates the critical path must represent all disciplines involved in the process. For example, a team developing a critical path for management of chemically dependent clients would likely include representatives of nursing, chemical dependency counselors, pharmacy, and social work services, as well as the clinical director. Another valuable perspective comes from clients and their families or caregivers. The team should elicit information from the people the process is designed to benefit. Similarly, if other parties are involved in the process, but are not team members, their input will also need to be elicited.

Creating the critical path. To progress, team members will need to reach consensus on the key activities involved in each stage of the care process. Members can draw on personal experience and knowledge, existing clinical literature and practice guidelines, and patient perspectives. Be assured that varying styles, methods, and approaches to care will arise in the team review. The resulting discussion can yield important knowledge about care delivery. If varied practice patterns are such that the group cannot reach consensus, the path should not dictate one approach over the other; separate paths can be developed when necessary. Over time the value of various critical paths can be evaluated empirically.

Remember also that the path need not be limited to clinical activities. A critical path could include addressing the need for provision of client management information as a prelude to discharge. Critical paths should also include outcomes.

Despite the complexity of the processes involved, teams should attempt to make their paths as concise as possible—one page is ideal—so ultimately they can be used as practical tools in daily practice.

The time needed to develop a critical path may vary from two hours to four months. Organizations should be prepared to invest a significant commitment of time and effort during the development cycle.

Typically critical paths will address many specific areas of care including

- consultations,
- tests,
- medications,
- treatments/interventions,
- nutrition,
- education,
- symptom control,
- discharge planning,
- psychosocial management, and
- expected outcomes.

Defining the care delivery outcomes that are expected during the episode of care covered by the critical path. Outcomes have become an increasingly important aspect of all individual-focused management activities, and this perspective is reflected in critical path development. The critical path design team determines what the patient is expected to achieve or be able to perform at specific intervals in the care plan.

Results. At all stages of the care process, staff, especially clinical staff, can refer to critical paths to guide decision making. They should be available to all involved personnel in all the relevant work areas and office locations. Critical paths are also valuable for clients; they can increase clients' knowledge of the care plan and sense of partnership with providers.

Examples of Improvement

▣ Example 5.1: Promoting Quality Care by Use of Critical Pathways and Care Plans

Note: In this example, a mental health provider undertook the development of a number of critical pathways for common psychiatric disorders. Its improvement approach was designed to satisfy both internal and external customers, including clients and their families, staff, and managed care organizations. Using this methodology, it improved individual case planning and also joined together for the first time system care planning with expected outcomes and clinical standards. The project also realized an important improvement by clinician tracking of client responses throughout their continuum of care, using a customized critical path/treatment plan format. The results overall also indicated care delivery documentation could be enhanced by detailing responses to treatment at critical junctures with desired outcomes using critical pathways.

Overhead and Opportunity

This example describes a hospital's effort to more effectively manage episodes of illness through a care planning process. This process grew out of the total quality management (TQM) approach within the hospital. It represented the hospital's positive response to the increasingly rigorous psychiatric utilization review and managed care pressure it was experiencing. But also, more proactively, the process represented an important shift in philosophy and delivery of care that was more responsive to the needs of clients and their families.

The process was developed by a multi-disciplinary team, including nurses, social workers, therapeutic recreation specialists, psychologists, and psychiatrists. The team spent significant time reviewing the literature and examining care mapping examples, and formulating and identifying an appropriate structure for the care planning tool. The early prototypes of the care planning process were based on acuity levels and patient characteristics. Later variations included more specific pathways for different age groups and served as models for long-term coordinated care planning.

There were also two important objectives associated with the care plan project. The first was to design a treatment plan that could be not only highly customized to diagnostic categories, but also highly reflective of an individual's clinical needs. As a prelude to this phase, the team developed materials linking diagnosis with problem statements, interventions, and outcome factors. It also developed a method to portray the plan in a graphic format, allowing for easy visualization.

A second related aspect of the care planning process allowed providers to document "detours" or critical moments when clients veered off the critical pathway. Detours are considered critically important to review in a treatment planning context and also provide feedback on the variability of client and pathway choice combinations.

The care planning process design specifications included one working document that would be used for all care providers with specific standards of care, blending treatment planning with the critical path tracking system. There was significant hope that such an approach would eliminate duplication of care by various providers, increase coordination among the treatment team, and provide a better documentation format to track detours and untoward patient events. Finally, the team believed that use of the care planning process would establish a much more cost-effective approach that would be attractive to third party payers. It was also anticipated that use of such a system would yield a much better database, linking clinical outcomes, diagnostic groups, and interventions, and would ultimately allow benchmarks to be set for length of stay.

Implementation

Care plans were developed for the most common and typical diagnoses presented to the system (for example, depressive disorders, anxiety disorders, personality disorders). Staff were fully trained in the use of the care plans and participated in a pilot project to evaluate the applicability and appropriateness of each plan.

The care planning process used a convenient approach to chart plan building. Staff selected problems from an existing list and documentation of problem areas included outcome criteria target dates and a dictionary of treatment interventions. The indicated service areas also required attached time frames and complementary quality measures to track delivery of care.

Outcomes

The hospital's care planning project resulted in a variety of positive outcomes:

- Overall length of stay was significantly reduced (by approximately eight days);
- Use of the guided pathways and charting of detours increased the accuracy, comprehensiveness, and clarity of documentation of exceptions in client care;

■ A significant amount of multi-disciplinary learning occurred, both in the development of the plans, the implementation of the plans, and the review of outcomes data associated with their use; and

■ The critical paths provided the facility a conceptual model to understand and link diagnostic categories with interventions and expected outcomes within time frames.

▣ Example 5-2: Use of Experimental Design Methods To Improve Patient Satisfaction with Care

Note: This is an interesting and advanced example of improvement methodologies in health care focusing on improving patient satisfaction with care. Highlights of the case example include the systematic and rigorous examination of potential interventions, care, and discipline to continue tracking over time, teasing apart causal factors, and use of a relatively advanced experimental methodology to make quality improvement efforts.

Opportunity

A large medical center recognized a problem with patient satisfaction in its emergency and urgent care services area. This service area provides both medical and psychiatric services. The center also realized that issues of patient satisfaction and compliance, behavioral management, and overall therapeutic milieu management were essential for quality emergency room service. Consumer surveys administered during the past three years indicated that the center's patients were significantly less satisfied than those of competing health care facilities.

Patient satisfaction was selected as an aspect of care targeted for improvement, although this initiative was also part of a larger TQM/continuous quality improvement (CQI) effort within the medical center.

Plan and Approach

A project improvement team was formed, involving numerous administrative and clinical leadership representatives and stakeholders (nurse manager, emergency room registration coordinator, staff nursing representative, mental health psychiatric assignment officer, surgical technician). A model for process improvement paralleling the plan-do-check-act cycle was selected as a way to approach the problem. The steps the team used for the design included 1) exploring of the feasibility of experimentation; 2) developing suggestions for possible clinical and administrative changes; 3) designing and implementing the overall experiment; 4) collecting the data to analyze the results and making conclusions; 5) making decisions based on those outcomes involving process changes where necessary; and 6) planning for future experimentation. Critical to the process of improvement are the decision making and process changes that follow the general approach described above.

The key outcome of interest for the project team focused on patient dissatisfaction with the emergency room. To begin, the team developed a measurement system focusing on discharge of patients from the emergency room. A random telephone survey was conducted daily with selected patients from the discharge logs. During the first phase of improvement, the team used traditional quality improvement techniques (for example, Pareto charts and scatter diagrams of waiting time and dissatisfaction). A detailed review of the findings suggested a common finding in assessment of emergency room waiting times (namely, that the "perception" of waiting is perhaps equal to, if not more important than, actual waiting time as related to satisfaction). The team continued its work, following traditional quality improvement activities, and implemented a change in physician scheduling that improved patient flow.

The team conducted a brainstorming session with key process owners, including physicians, nurses, ancillary staff, and current and former patients. The brainstorming session focused on ideas that might increase patients' satisfaction within the emergency room. A comprehensive list was made and the team narrowed the ideas to factors they considered feasible, cost-effective, and practical. Throughout this process, administrative and clinical leadership kept the focus of the project on practical, feasible, pragmatic changes that would have impact. The team planned the experiment and considered options for each factor that included several process modifications (for example, fast track to service, internal operations modifications, triage area changes, outside waiting room changes, pediatric changes). The factors were identified and corresponding changes (minus and plus) were considered. An initial experiment was determined, which included a variety of changes (for example, fast track offered to non-emergency patients, registered nurse follow-up after the day of discharge, pamphlets in the triage area, and staff providing coloring books and crayons to pediatric patients).

Outcome

Following detailed data collection, patient satisfaction data was plotted over time and the team discovered that the combination of use of a fast track and overall pediatric changes significantly reduced patients' dissatisfaction. The team reasoned that the combination of changes particularly helped pediatric patients become more satisfied, which in turn satisfied the adult caregivers and caretakers who accompanied children to the emergency room.

The team was particularly pleased that the combination of services provided better services to the different sets of patients. Following the experiment, the team recommended implementing the fast track system and making final changes to the pediatric treatment room. To continue to track and monitor the outcome and performance of the process, the team maintained control charts to show the ongoing satisfaction/dissatisfaction rates.

Summary

This project team, working in a large medical center, produced an extraordinary change in its emergency room service satisfaction rates. Several key outcomes emerged from the projects, including 1) a good example of process improvement application in a health care setting; 2) recognition that statistical understanding can be shared among managers, clinicians, and quality experts; 3) recognition of understanding that delivery of care is multidimensional and multifaceted in its nature and as such may require more complex designs to assess outcomes of change; and 4) the importance of continuing to look for a combination of interventions that may add up to more than their individual contributions (for example, developing the fast track and pediatric changes at the same time).

▣ Chapter Summary
What Are the Goals of Improvement?

- Continued improvement, not "optimal" performance;
- Specific, measurable improvements for identified dimensions of performance;

- Improvements that are measurable and sustainable; and
- Improvements that target processes, but address any problems associated with individual clinicians or staff.

Who Takes Improvement Actions?

- The process' owners, customers, and suppliers design and test improvements.
- The organization's leaders approve changes that involve significant resources or effects.
- Changes should be explained in an educational, nonthreatening way to all people who carry out the process.

How Do We Improve Processes?

- Use a systematic method to plan, test, assess, and fully implement the changes.
- Use qualitative and quantitative tools, including multivoting, selection grids, cause-and-effect diagrams, run charts, flowcharts, and histograms.
- Use critical paths to design new processes or redesign existing processes.

▣ References

Bower KA: Developing and using critical paths. In Lord JT (ed): *The Physician Leader's Guide*. Rockville, MD: Bader & Associates, Inc, pp 61–66, 1992.

Dunn J, Rodriguez D, Novak JJ: Promoting quality mental health care delivery with critical care path care plans. *J Psychosoc Nurs Ment Health Serv* 32(7):25–29, 1994.

Moore CH: Experimental design in healthcare. *Quality Management in Health Care* 2(2):13–26, 1994.

Weber DO: Clinical pathways stretch patient care but shrink costly lengths of stay at Anne Arundel Medical Center in Annapolis, Maryland. *Strateg Health Excell* 5(5):1–11, 1992.

Zander K: Critical pathways. In Melum MM, Sinioris MK (eds): *Total Quality Management: The Health Care Pioneers*. Chicago: American Hospital Publishing, Inc, pp 305–314, 1992.

6

Case Studies

"It seems a helluva note in life that we must pay a dealer to be nice to his customers."

—Lee Iacocca, commenting on a new Chrysler policy of giving bigger factory rebates to dealerships that earn better customer service ratings, in *Training*

- Case Studies
- References

This chapter presents two examples illustrating the performance improvement cycle that are adapted from actual experiences in behavioral health care organizations. The examples show the variety of performance improvement approaches and the wide range of processes that can be improved. They also illustrate the varying complexity of improvement activities. Equally important, the tenacity, teamwork, and creativity evident in these examples should create enthusiasm for the possibilities inherent in the framework for improving performance. They also demonstrate the value of a comprehensive, systematic approach to quality improvement.

Case Studies

◨ **Example 6-1: Improving State-Funded Child Psychiatric Care: Reducing Extended Hospitalizations Through Changes in Treatment Planning**

Source: Adapted from Mossman D, et al: Improving state-funded child psychiatric care: reducing protracted hospitalizations through challenges in treatment planning. *Qual Rev Bull* 16(1):20–24, 1990. Reprinted with permission.

Opportunity and the Setting

This example is about a state-funded psychiatric center for children in a hospital setting serving children 5 to 17 years of age. The majority of the children are poor, and many have been placed in the custody of community agencies (for example, county Departments of Human Services). The center operates under political and financial constraints that differ from those affecting private psychiatric facilities. At the same time, its client demographics and treatment philosophy reflect changing professional attitudes about psychiatric inpatient care.

In late 1986, the center's medical and social work staff recognized that the length of hospitalization for many children lasted beyond their individual needs for such intensive treatments. The average length of stay (LOS) was well over 100 days. Some children stayed for months awaiting residential placement; others remained in the hospital because of a lack of appropriate community services or delays in arranging appropriate aftercare services. The center anticipated that changes in several hospital practices would reduce extended hospitalizations. This example describes several of the center's changes in discharge planning and treatment and the effects of those changes on lengthy hospitalizations.

Changes in Treatment Process and Discharge Planning

Following a period of review, study, and planning, the center initiated a number of changes targeted at shortening the LOS for children. These included the following:

- The staff devised new comprehensive individual treatment plan forms requiring that a projected discharge date be set within 10 days of admission. Previously, such a date was not established until a child was judged ready for discharge. This was an important initiative because outside agencies often could not engage in any actual discharge planning or make appropriate referrals until a specific date had been established. Setting a discharge date shortly after admission allowed all parties involved with the child's care to begin discharge planning early in hospitalization.

- The discharge date was reviewed at regular treatment planning meetings. The change allowed for re-estimation of the planned discharge (for example, if the child needed more hospital treatment than first anticipated). Also, children could be discharged before the original date if follow-up was arranged and their in-hospital treatment needs had been met.

- The center also established a policy of remaining committed to the discharge date if the child was judged clinically ready for discharge. Previous policy had allowed hospitalization to continue simply because permanent placement was not available. Under the new policy, if permanent dispositions had not been arranged by the discharge date, children were to be discharged to an interim placement where they would await transfer to a residential facility.

■ With increased emphasis on prompt discharge planning, the center assigned a high priority to the paperwork needed to secure residential or foster care for children unable to return home following their hospitalizations.

■ To facilitate review, the center developed a new format for sending out reports to help speed release of records to agencies that reviewed materials for placement and to agencies providing follow-up care.

■ The center's social workers were expected to work closely with caseworkers from the Department of Human Services, juvenile court, and other social service agencies in planning for discharge. The social workers kept other agencies' representatives apprised of treatment progress. Outside representatives were invited to the treatment team meetings so that conjoint planning could occur, and were contacted if they did not attend. At times, supervisors were contacted if the caseworkers could not work out interagency problems. The center's social workers closely followed outside agencies' planning efforts, and supervisors were contacted if the discharge process was delayed unnecessarily.

■ The social work department worked closely with local community mental health centers (CMHCs) to smooth the referral process. Contracts between the center and the community agencies were reviewed at quarterly meetings of the hospital social workers and agency liaisons, and new agreements were reached regarding notice of referral for aftercare.

- The center's social work department increased the intensity of family therapy services offered to clients and their families. This effort focused on allowing children either to be discharged sooner or to return home, instead of going to a residential placement since unresolved family issues often prevented children from being discharged.

- Through meetings and phone conversations with various court personnel, the center's physicians and social workers outlined, in detail, the referral process and hospital admission criteria. These criteria helped probate and juvenile courts better understand what type of psychiatric disorders are treated appropriately in a hospital and what type of services the center provides. Courts were also encouraged to refer children for psychiatric evaluation, rather than simply order a child to the hospital. The center anticipated that this would eliminate admission of children who posed dispositional problems or who did not need hospital care, keep admission and treatment decisions within the purview of treatment teams, and keep discharge and LOS linked to clinical issues rather than to arbitrary time frames or external factors. Courts were also informed that children who did not meet inpatient admission criteria could not stay at the center simply because they had nowhere else to go.

- The psychiatry staff also have taken a more active stand regarding children who are committed involuntarily to the center. For example, psychiatrists increased their use of the Notice of Discharge form, which informs courts of the upcoming discharge of children who either were committed inappropriately or whose term of commitment has exceeded their need for hospital treatment.

Assessments

As part of a comprehensive assessment impact, a concurrent study of factors affecting LOS at the center was undertaken. These data indicated that diagnosis, age, and sex influence LOS, although several other factors (including history of criminal involvement, sexual and physical abuse, substance abuse, previous hospitalization, living situation, previous foster or residential placement, and parental divorce or work history) do not. The center compared the diagnosis, age, and sex distributions of children over time (before and after the changes) to assess whether variations in these areas could account for variation in LOS. Finally, the readmission rates over time were examined to help gauge whether more expeditious discharges resulted in an increased likelihood that a child would be rehospitalized within six months.

Outcomes

A number of findings emerged:

- The center's community-focused efforts yielded shorter hospitalizations and fewer extended hospital stays.
- Evidence for stable readmission rates over time supports the conviction that shorter hospitalizations did not lead to poorer services.
- Although it is difficult to quantify, a distinct improvement was noted in the CMHC's abilities to provide appointments for children and their families during the first week following discharge.

■ A recognition that the center's revised treatment policies affected not only LOS, but also the institution's relationship with and perception in the community. Because the center's social workers were very conscientious about giving outside agencies notice of discharge dates, those agencies, in general, became more responsive to children's needs for timely placement.

▣ Example 6-2: A Quality Improvement Effort Within Chemical Dependency: Treatment Planning and Relapse

Source: Adapted from Weedman R: *QI and Relapse Prevention.* Naples, FL: Healthcare Network, Inc, 1993. Reprinted with permission.

Background

A 45-bed residential and intensive outpatient treatment center provides services to adult psychoactive substance abusers. The center has a total of 62 staff, including a medical director, a consulting psychiatrist, a licensed graduate degree clinical coordinator, registered nurses, and certified addiction counselors with a range of education from high school degrees to graduate degrees in counseling and other health care sciences.

The center uses a biopsychosocial approach to treatment with the goal of assisting the client in arresting his or her addiction and maintaining ongoing abstinence and sobriety through the use of self-help fellowships.

Assessment

The faculty initiated a quality improvement process focusing, in part, on treatment of addiction problems and dynamics of relapse. Three initial steps included the following:

- *Giving authority equal to responsibility.* The center's performance improvement (PI) committee is responsible for and has authority over facility-wide monitoring, evaluation, and performance improvement activities.
- *Delineation of scope of care and service.* The facility provides comprehensive biopsychosocial residential and intensive outpatient assessment and treatment to adult psychoactive substance abusers.
- *Identification of important aspects of care and service.* Individualized residential treatment is tailored to address addiction problems and prevent relapse behaviors.

These initial efforts were followed by indicator development targeted on treatment and relapse prevention.

Indicator 1: Clients understand the dynamics of their relationship with the progressive nature of their psychoactive substance use disorder.

Threshold: 80%

Collection of Data: Performance evaluation clerk reviews 100% of client records three days prior to discharge to check if the progress notes reflect the attainment of treatment objectives that address the client's understanding of his or her addiction.

Indicator 2: Clients develop continuing care plans to address the dynamics of their identified relapse stressors and/or identified relapse behaviors.

Threshold: 80%

Collection of Data: Performance evaluation clerk reviews 100% of client records three days prior to discharge to check if the progress notes reflect the attainment of treatment objectives that address the client's plans to address his/her identified relapse stressors/behaviors.

Indicator 3: Clients maintain abstinence from mood-altering chemicals for six months post discharge from residential treatment.

Threshold: 65%

Collection of Data: Continuing care coordinator tracks 20 discharges monthly from the residential service. Follow-up tracking is conducted through a telephone interview with the client and an identified client associate six months post discharge.

Clients' Understanding of Addiction and Treatment Planning

Data Collection and Evaluation Findings (Indicators 1 and 2). Record reviews for the first quarter (36 records) revealed that 52% of the clients did not understand the dynamics of their relationship with the progressive nature of their psychoactive substance use disorder. The average length of stay for the first quarter was 17.6 days.

A review of the last quarter of the previous year (42 records) revealed that 56% of the clients also did not understand the dynamics of their relationship with the progressive nature of their psychoactive substance use disorder. Consistently, therefore, a com-pliance average of approximately 52% has been maintained with this indicator.

Data from the first quarter indicated no change in the average score. Analysis of this pattern suggests that the lack of threshold compliance in the adult residential service suggested the following:

- The psychoactive use assessments are not clearly reflecting the severity of the client's pathological relationship with psychoactive substances.
- Treatment plans inadequately address the client's defeating relationship with alcohol and other drugs.
- Progress notes inadequately reflect the client's positive response to treatment relative to his/her understanding the dynamics of the relationship with alcohol/drugs.

A review of demographic profiles of the clients did not yield correlation between understanding and age or sex of the clients, the drug of choice, the need for detoxification services, or any specific clinicians assigned to clients. However, length of stay and understanding were related. For example, it was noted that in 100% of the cases reviewed, none of the clients in treatment for less than nine days understood the dynamics of their relationship with psychoactive substances.

Explanation of Root Causes and Team Building. The center's PI committee recognized that there were most likely multiple causes to the problem of clients not understanding the dynamics of their addiction, including

- possible inappropriate placement of clients at a given level of care;
- the lack of a process yielding a substantive clinical assessment of the client;
- counseling staff's inadequate clinical skills to specifically assess the client's dynamics of addiction;
- inadequate knowledge and limited technical competence among clinical staff to formulate an individualized treatment plan; and
- deficiencies in individual and group counseling skills to enhance clients' understandings of the dynamics of their addictions.

The PI committee also recognized that this process (that is, helping clients enhance their understanding of addiction) involves both clinical and support staff. Following this thinking, they formed a quality action team with a medical records clerk, a nurse, a physician, and two counselors.

The quality council helped further define the project to be addressed by the quality action team and helped the team draft a planning statement.

The plan consisted of

- identification of the facilitator-consultant;
- identification of the team leader-counselor;
- identification of team members;
- definition of expected outcomes (for example, to identify causes of the problems and implement a corrective action plan within six months; and
- definition of specific outcomes (for example, 70% of the clients are to understand the dynamics of their defeating relationship with psychoactive substance use disorders).

Actions Taken to Improve Care. The actions taken by the quality improvement team consisted of the following:

- The process of refining the admission assessment to evaluate the severity of the presenting problems was redesigned to ensure that with few exceptions, the admission criteria for residential care were met.
- The medical interpretations relative to the history and physical examination were changed to highlight the findings relative to the presenting problems and chemical dependency.
- Addiction assessments were revised to effectively capture the severity of addiction, the patterns, the circumstances, and the effects of use.
- In-service training was conducted to educate all disciplines in writing measurable treatment objectives that more specifically assessed the client's understanding of the dynamics of his/her addiction.

Continued Monitoring. Staff-specific recommendations were monitored by the clinical coordinator and the PI committee continued to monitor overall outcomes including the staff-specific recommendations.

Communication of Results. Copies of the overall analysis were shared with the staff at the semi-annual professional staff organization meeting. Aggregate findings continued to be summarized by the service review committee and were included in the regular quarterly quality improvement report distribution.

Relapse Prevention

Evaluation of Findings (Indicator 3). Data collected from the continuing care coordinator that evaluated the abstinence of clients who were discharged the first two quarters (103 clients) revealed that 48% maintained abstinence from all mood-altering chemicals for a period of six months post discharge. The established threshold was that 65% of the clients would be expected to maintain abstinence; therefore, the findings were well under the established threshold.

It was noted that for those clients who relapsed, none of the clients' records provided evidence that they "understood relapse stressors" by the time of discharge. However, for all of the clients discharged for the study in question, only 12% of clients could identify stressors that might trigger drug-seeking behaviors and relapse.

It was also noted that in all records reviewed, only 12% of the records clearly defined stressors in the client's life. Additionally, only 12% of the treatment plans related to the treatment of stressors in the client's life.

Analysis of this pattern suggested the following:

- The psychoactive use assessments did not clearly reflect the severity of the client's pathological relationship with psychoactive substances.
- Treatment plans inadequately addressed the client's defeating relationship with alcohol and other drugs, and failed to identify relapse stressors.

- Treatment consistently did not adequately address the client's need for a social support system; or identify work-related problems, methods of dealing with anger or boredom, or methods of coping with family stressors.
- Progress notes inadequately reflected the client's positive response to treatment relative to understanding the dynamics of the relationship with alcohol/drugs.

Exploration of Root Causes and Team Building. The center's PI committee recognized the multidimensional nature of relapse and the contributions to abstinence for a period of six months post treatment. Key factors included

- a limited ability to conduct substantive clinical assessment of the client that identified relapse stressors;
- limited clinical skills on the part of counselors to assess the clients' dynamics of addiction or address relapse stressors;
- inadequate knowledge and limited technical competence among clinical staff to formulate an individualized treatment plan to address relapse stressors; and
- deficiencies in individual and group counseling skills to enhance clients' understandings of the dynamics of their addiction and relapse stressors.

Similar to the earlier quality effort, the PI committee formed a multiprofessional quality team with a counselor from the intensive outpatient program, a consulting psychiatrist, two counselors, and a consulting relapse prevention specialist.

The quality council helped further define the project to be addressed by the quality action team.

The plan consisted of

- identification of the facilitator-consultant;
- identification of the team leader-counselor;
- identification of team members;
- definition of expected outcomes (for example, to identify causes of the problems and implement a corrective action plan within six months); and
- definition of specific outcomes (for example, 60% of the clients are to be able to maintain abstinence from the use of psychoactive substances for a period of six months post treatment).

Actions Taken to Improve Care. The actions taken by the QI team consisted of the following:

- Develop a cause-and-effect diagram to identify the customers and processes of care that are involved in relapse prevention (referring agent, admissions, counseling staff, outpatient counselors, employers, family, social support [friends], and external case managers).
- Discussion about possible corrective actions with workshop participants relative to care processes.

▣ References

Mossman D, et al: Improving state funded child psychiatric care: Reducing protracted hospitalizations through changes in treatment planning. *Qual Rev Bull* 16(1):20–24, 1990.

Weedman R: *QI and Relapse Prevention.* Naples, FL: Healthcare Network, Inc, 1993.

Appendix

A

A Primer on Behavioral Health Care Outcomes Measures

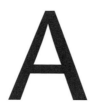 **Overview**

The principal goal of behavioral health care is improvement of client outcomes. All of health care is rapidly moving from an era of managed care toward an era of managed outcomes and disease management approaches. Outcomes thinking in behavioral health care emphasizes the end results of providing care to the consumer of the services. Outcomes evaluation also includes the collection, aggregation, and analysis of data relevant to quality assessment and improvement.

Concerns over spiraling costs of care have increased the need for reliable data about care outcomes. Increasingly, there are also strong forces directing public reporting of information of health systems' performance. There is also significant belief that improved methods and use of outcomes research in care delivery will lead to reduced costs and improved quality.

To begin to effectively evaluate behavioral health care, two broad requirements are needed: 1) a definition of outcomes and 2) appropriate measures to assess outcomes. While these issues appear straightforward, they are not.

Behavioral health care affects the whole person in a complex process. Consider for a moment the complexities involved in assessing processes and outcomes for a single outpatient group psychotherapy encounter or effectiveness of treatment over time. From an evaluation standpoint, the leadership style and effectiveness of leaders, effects from the group milieu, any adverse consequences of the session, the cost of the treatment, the client's perception of service, and the client's clinical status would be evaluated. A comprehensive outcomes approach might also provide information relevant to the nine dimensions of performance (that is, efficacy, appropriateness, availability, timeliness, effectiveness, continuity, safety, efficiency, and respect and caring).

Until recently, the outcomes of behavioral health care services have been primarily oriented toward assessment of psychopathology (particularly symptom duration and severity) and utilization (particularly length of stay and readmission rates). In the last several years, a much broader perspective has begun to develop that includes a wider range of outcomes for the individual, family, workplace, and community.

This appendix provides a beginning definition of outcomes, explores some of the methodological and substantive issues surrounding measurement of care outcomes, and briefly reviews some of the available measures applicable to behavioral health care and related outcomes.

▣ Behavioral Health Care Outcomes: A Working Definition

Establishing a modest consensus on what we mean by outcomes is important. Outcomes can be defined "as states or conditions of individuals and populations attributed or attributable to antecedent health care. They include changes in health states, changes in knowledge or behavior pertinent to future health states, and satisfaction with health care (expressed as opinion or inferred from behavior)." (*Qual Rev Bull* 18(11):356, 1992.)

Or, to quote the earlier published Institute of Medicine Report commenting on quality and outcomes, "Quality of care is the degree to which health care services for individuals and populations increase the likelihood of desired health outcomes and are commensurate with current professional knowledge." (*Medicare: A Strategy for Quality Assurance, Vol 1.* Washington, DC: National Academy Press, p 21, 1990.)

These definitions of quality focus on health outcomes within the limitations of the current state of the art of medical knowledge.

To summarize, behavioral health care outcomes may include

- changes in mental health status,
- changes in knowledge and behavior pertinent to future mental health statutes, and
- satisfaction with care.

▣ Outcome Perspectives

More specifically, it is important to understand the effects of particular types of care received by a variety of clients with particular behavioral health problems. These issues and related questions, so relevant to health care discussions today, were raised cogently early in psychotherapy evaluation and research. For example, "What kinds of therapeutic procedures will be helpful to particular patients under particular circumstances?" (Strupp and Bergin, 1969; Bergin and Strupp, 1972).

In addition to understanding specific effects of specific treatments, outcomes considerations should also take into account short- and long-term

155

effects, traditional assessment of mortality and morbidity, and specific evaluations of mental health symptomatology, mental well being, capacity for work and function, and overall health-related quality of life.

Classic measures of outcomes in health care have generally included death, disease, disability, discomfort, and dissatisfaction—although their contrapositive concepts have become increasingly studied as well: survival, health, capability, comfort, and satisfaction.

Building on these broad measures and in accordance with existing research and clinical experience, more specific assessment of behavioral health care outcomes might include the following:

- Clinical variables;
- Biological and physiological assessments;
- Specific symptom measures;
- Physical, medical, and functional status;
- Personal adjustment;
- Quality of life, particularly health-related quality of life;
- Social and psychosocial features;
- Work capability and capacity;
- Risk of reoccurrence of symptoms/disease-relapse;
- Satisfaction and experience with care;
- Disability days—lost work days and/or interruption of activities of daily living;
- Longevity;
- Morbidity and mortality experience;
- Personal health and illness management;
- Self-efficacy;
- Cost of care/benefits of care; and
- Reports of family and/or significant others.

These more specific outcomes measures can be interwoven with the nine dimensions of performance to create a conceptual map to guide measurement activities (see Figure A–1, page 157).

Examples of Specific Behavioral Outcomes Assessments

Dimensions of Performance	Examples of Specific Behavioral Outcomes Assessments				
	Symptoms	Quality of Life	Biological/ Medical	Self-Efficacy	Cost
Efficacy	�				
Appropriateness					▢
Availability		▢			
Timeliness			▢		
Effectiveness					
Continuity		▢			
Safety				▢	
Efficiency					▢
Respect and Caring	▢	▢			

Figure A–1 ■ *This figure illustrates a conceptual map to guide measurement activities.*

Any combination of outcomes assessments could be paired with the dimensions of performance, depending on the relevance of the measure to the performance concept and the organizational functions under review.

Another relevant perspective regarding outcomes emerges from the National Institute of Mental Health (NIMH) National Plan (1989), which highlights recommendations regarding the scope and priorities of behavioral health services research. The NIMH National Plan identifies the five following major areas of concern:

Epidemiology. What are the characteristics of those seeking behavioral health services, including their demographics, risk factors, cultural influences, and family issues?

Assessment. What are the best means to assess a person's physical, psychological, social, and vocational disabilities or functioning?

Treatment. What are the best methods of estimating the effectiveness of treatment services of varying complexities and in different settings tailored to specific target populations?

Rehabilitation and habilitation. What are the best methods of estimating the effectiveness of rehabilitative services to improve or support social skills, capacity for independent living, or vocational rehabilitation?

Outcomes. What are the best methods for estimating the impact of behavioral health care services within and across four outcomes domains— clinical symptoms, social and vocational functioning, humanitarian sense of well-being for the consumer and family, and public welfare benefits?

▣ Methodological Issues and Outcomes as Quality Measures

It is likely that outcomes evaluations will continue to advance down two broad paths: 1) traditional, randomized clinical trials of therapeutic efficacy and evaluations in clinical laboratories, and 2) specific evaluations within the everyday care practice. In many organizations, outcomes information is being collected on a routine basis as care is delivered. Such information has become part of daily exchanges between managed care organizations and care providers (for example, Does current psychiatric status match level of care? What is the expected length of stay based on current response to treatment?).

The use of outcome measures for quality of care indicators has some special methodological issues that are worth reviewing. Some general evaluation issues include the following:

- Recruitment and use of adequate numbers of clients;
- Defining the population to be studied;
- Defining the treatments to be studied;
- Controlling treatment-related effects;
- Establishing appropriate comparison and control groups;
- Assessing treatment bias of clients and staff;

- Conducting appropriate follow-ups;
- Use of process and structural analysis;
- Appropriate time windows for measurement;
- Usefulness and understandability of data;
- Quality of performance;
- Cause-and-effect relationships between process and outcomes;
- Case-mix adjustment;
- Understanding the nature of outcomes as integrative;
- Costs/benefits of data; and
- Use of outcomes norms.

Available Measures

Many different measures are available to assess care outcomes, including assessment of symptomatology, general functioning, social adjustment, quality of life, and psychophysiological factors affecting pain, function, and disability. There are also client satisfaction measures in behavioral health care. Various assessment devices represent a set of measures that have demonstrated validity, reliability, and relative ease of application in a clinical setting.

◉ **Example A-1: An Outcome Monitoring System for Psychiatric Care**

Source: Adapted from Stevenson JF, et al: An outcome monitoring system of psychiatric inpatient care. *Qual Rev Bull* 14:326–331, 1988. Reprinted with permission.

Note: This is an example of one hospital's efforts to convert a set of research-oriented outcomes measures into a practical, clinically relevant monitoring system. Organizations interested in developing or implementing an outcomes monitoring system may be able to learn from the problems confronted and solutions attempted at this hospital. Thus far, it appears that the information generated by the outcome monitoring system can be used to meet the hospital's original objectives. Collection of such data over longer periods of time with more patients will greatly enhance the value of this outcome monitoring system and provide an essential empirical platform for future quality improvements.

Introduction

This example describes a system for monitoring psychiatric inpatient outcomes that was implemented at a 108-bed psychiatric hospital. This technically sophisticated system relies on patient interview data gathered using several established assessment instruments during the care process. Through interviews, patient problems prior to admission are identified and, in some cases, the degree of impairment is rated. Following discharge, patients' levels of impairment and improvement are rated. Ideally, by implementing this system on an ongoing basis, a behavioral health care organization can identify trends in patient problems, as well as areas where more favorable outcomes (for example, a lower rate of patient readmissions) may be obtained through specific improvements in care.

System Development and Background

The outcomes monitoring system described in this example grew out of a grant to study the problem-oriented record system. Study researchers developed a battery of outcomes measures in order to gather outcomes data needed to evaluate the system.

The outcomes data produced by the study reflected favorably on the hospital's care and was later included in the department of evaluation's (DOE's) annual report. After evaluating these data, hospital administrators enthusiastically supported developing a cost-effective outcomes monitoring system for use on an ongoing basis. The DOE system was designed to:

- Provide data for internal hospital program evaluation;
- Support and enhance grant proposals and research projects conducted with patients; and
- Generate studies and reports that would add to the literature on psychiatric outcomes monitoring.

Patient interviews provide the primary data source for this monitoring system, with supplemental background information abstracted from medical records. A baseline interview conducted during the patient's stay gathers information on patient functioning during the month prior to admission. This initial interview is conducted at a computer terminal located off the treatment ward. Two follow-up interviews are also conducted: one by telephone at 1 month post-discharge and another 12 months after admission.

Implementation

The DOE hired an interviewer with prior experience as a behavioral health care worker to conduct most of the interview activities required by the outcomes monitoring system. The interviewer's experience was invaluable in helping him to be as responsive as possible to the needs of both patients and health care professionals at the hospital.

In the initial phase, a 5% random sample of newly admitted patients, selected daily, was included in the five-month study. This sample would have amounted to approximately 130 patients per year. Patients discharged within three days were dropped from the sample and replaced. A "tracking file" was created for each patient selected for monitoring. All personnel working with these patients (for example, nursing staff and the attending physician) were informed of the patient's involvement in the study by means of a standard note attached to the patient's chart.

The interviewer's first task was to set up a patient's baseline interview three days after the patient was admitted. (The hospital's average length of stay is approximately 15 days.) At that point, the interviewer consulted the patient's chart and the nursing staff to ascertain the patient's readiness to be interviewed. Many patients still experienced severe symptoms at that point and could not be interviewed. For such cases, the interviewer would monitor each patient's chart to determine when the patient was ready for an interview. Such refusals were viewed as temporary; few patients were unwilling to be interviewed for the entire length of their inpatient stay.

Of the 37 patients selected for inclusion in the pilot study, 27 (73%) were actually interviewed. Reasons for loss from the sample included discharge on short notice or against medical advice, prohibitively severe symptoms up to the time of discharge, and patient refusal.

Patients participating in the pilot study were hospitalized an average of 9 days prior to their interview, with a range from 6–15 days.

Outcome

Twenty-seven baseline and 23 one-month follow-up interviews were conducted, representing an 85% follow-up rate of the original group. Although the sample was small, it serves to demonstrate that the system produces meaningful outcomes data and provides an emerging examination of the pattern of patient outcomes and relationships between them.

The baseline interview data indicated that depression, anxiety, and difficulties with anger or irritability were the most frequent self-reported problems in the month prior to admission. When major problems are aggregated into seven subscales, mood and social behavior problems were most common. The greatest patient-rated improvement level was in reduction of overt behavioral systems, whereas the lowest level of improvement was reported in problems with life tasks (for example, work and school-related activities). The most significant findings note improvements in depression/anxiety and grandiosity/externalization. Although the frequency of self-perceived positive mood states increased following treatment, the frequency of undesirable social behavior remained constant. Interviewer-rated global functioning also increased markedly.

Over time, as the internal database accumulates, the outcomes monitoring system is anticipated to have a number of applications, including the following:

■ Such data could be used to compare discharge plans and actual post-discharge experience. Ideally, such comparisons would produce indicators of rehospitalization and identify unmet aftercare needs.

- The DOE plans to compare monitoring data with computerized medical record information for internal consistency (for example, data from the mental status examination completed by a physician upon admission).

- In addition to estimating overall effectiveness of hospital treatment, the DOE plans to compare and contrast subcategories of patients by diagnosis or major problems.

- Changes in case mix over time can also be examined and alternate treatments for the same problem can be compared in a quasi-experimental design.

- These data also hold promise for generalization of treatment and aftercare planning prospectively for patients with similar diagnoses undergoing similar treatments.

▣ Appendix Summary

Given the information on care outcomes currently available, and knowledge gained from outcomes research more broadly, a number of recommendations stand out as worthy of note.

Outcome Guidelines

- Use available, existing measures in literature.
- Incorporate outcomes measures into systematic, ongoing, and longitudinal assessment of quality assurance and continuous quality improvement programs.
- Compare health care provider and program data to existing data in the local community and, when possible, to the national experience.
- Use every opportunity to capture outcome data.
- Employ specific performance dimensions and associated measures that are relevant and salient to the organization, the situation of

care, the characteristics of the patients, and the structure, process, and outcomes of care.

- Acknowledge the inherent complexity in the interrelations of structure, process, and outcomes in clinical settings.

- Expand the understanding of outcomes to other "customers" in the health care settings and examine the relationship between outcomes assessments of key customers such as physicians and clients.

- Consider that future client experience and outcomes assessment will likely include more point-of-service data, telecommunication exchanges, video and multimedia assessment systems, and broad evaluations of not only problems, but the goodness of aspects of care, the personal acceptability of care, and other customer perspectives using state-of-the art management information systems.

▣ References

Bergin, AE, Strupp HH: *Changing Frontiers in the Science of Psychotherapy.* Chicago: Aldine-Atherton, 1972.

National Institute of Mental Health: *The Future of Mental Health Services Research* (DHHS Publication No. ADM 89-1600). Washington, DC: U.S. Government Printing Office, 1989.

National Institute of Mental Health: *Caring for People With Severe Mental Disorders: A National Plan of Research to Improve Services* (DHHS Publication No. ADM 91-1762). Washington, DC: U.S. Government Printing Office, 1991.

Phelan M, Wykes T, Goldman H: Global function scales. *Soc Psychiatry Psychiatr Epidemiol* 29:205–211, 1994.

Ruggeri M: Patients' and relatives' satisfaction with psychiatric services: The state of the art of its measurement. *Soc Psychiatry Psychiatr Epidemiol* 29:212–227, 1994.

Stevenson JF, et al: An outcome monitoring system for psychiatric inpatient care. *Qual Rev Bull* 14:326–331, 1988.

Strupp HH, Bergin AE: Some empirical and conceptual bases for coordinated research in psychotherapy: A critical review of issues, trends, and evidence. *Int J Psychiatry* 7:18–90, 1969.

Appendix

B

Optimizing Teams and Teamwork

This appendix contains information about effective teamwork that should prove invaluable to advisory boards, organizational management, project staff, and any other groups involved in community-wide self-assessment and improvement. This information is taken, in part, from *Using Quality Improvement Tools in a Health Care Setting,* published by the Joint Commission.

▣ Introduction
Committees, Committees, Committees . . .

How often have we heard or made the statement, "I like my work, but I hate the meetings"? or "If I only had time to see my clients or get the real work done!" Most people have experienced the frustration of committees—their purpose is unclear, meetings ramble, one member dominates the discussion, no one speaks up, the chairperson is too dogmatic or offers no direction, turf battles dominate discussions, no one has the necessary expertise or the necessary data, everyone believes he or she has the answer but no one listens to each other, the group cannot reach consensus even about meeting dates and times, members are consistently late or absent. . . . The unhappy list seems to go on forever.

To eliminate some of these problems, eliminate the word *committee* for purposes of this discussion. *Committee* implies a permanent body with a broad, static purpose. Instead, use the word *team,* the term commonly employed for quality improvement. Teams are a vital part of behavioral health care practice, including clinical teams, quality teams, and special focus team. *Team* implies a group working together for a well-defined purpose. It also implies a group that will not be together forever, a particularly bleak and tiring aspect of some committees. Indeed, once a specific project or a series of projects is completed, a team often disbands—with a positive sense of accomplishment.

This appendix examines ground rules, team stages, and roles, and surveys some of the ingredients of a successful team. The overriding purpose of this discussion is to avoid the traps of a dysfunctional group described in the first paragraph.

▣ Teams

Teams need structure and support and time to grow. Do not expect a team to function at peak efficiency at the first or at every subsequent meeting. Like any group of people, the members of the improvement team must go through many stages in its life cycle. These stages include various mixtures of work and productivity.

Establishing major team tasks includes

- selecting the team,
- setting group rules,

- doing the groundwork,
- conducting team meetings and tracking outcomes, and
- completing the task.

Ground Rules: Begin at the Beginning

Setting the ground rules at the outset can help a team avoid endless distractions and detours on the route to improvement. Look at the ground rules as an opportunity to design a framework that allows the team to function smoothly. These typically include:

Decision making. The group must decide what kind of consensus or majority is needed for a decision, recognizing that decisions belong to the entire team.

Attendance. Attendance is crucial. Constant late arrivals and absences can sabotage the team's efforts. Set guidelines for attendance and hold to them.

Meeting schedule. For high attendance and steady progress, the team should agree on a regular time, day, and place for meetings. Also, the team should determine the frequency of meetings. These matters should be revisited at various times during the team's life.

Opportunity to speak. By agreeing at the outset to give all members an opportunity to contribute and to be heard with respect, the team will focus its attention on the important area of open communication.

Disagreements. The team must openly agree to disagree. It must acknowledge and accept that members will openly debate differences in viewpoint. It is fine for discussions to overflow outside the meeting room, but members should never feel that what they say in the hallway cannot be said in the meeting.

Assignments. The team should agree to complete assignments within the particular time limits so that delayed work from an individual does not delay the group.

Other rules. The team should discuss all other rules that members feel are important. These can include whether senior management staff should attend, whether pocket pagers should be checked at the door, what the break frequency is, and so forth.

▣ Team Roles

A team should function within a framework that will provide for its mission, support its activities through various resources, furnish it with reporting channels, and give it authority. This framework, in part, takes the form of roles for team members. Fulfilling these roles is necessary if a team is to progress steadily in its efforts.

Team Leader (Facilitator)

The team leader may be established before the rest of the team forms or may be selected at the first team meeting. Even if a team leader is designated before the team forms, the role of facilitating the meetings can be taken by another team member and may be changed several times during the project, or even during a single meeting. The facilitator's role is to be objective and to move the team along.

No matter who takes the baton, the team leader/facilitator must fulfill these essential duties:

- *Keep the discussion moving forward within the allotted time frame.* A sagging, digressing discussion can ruin forward momentum, adversely affect morale, hurt the leader's image, and put the team behind schedule. The leader should keep the discussion moving by containing digression, getting input from a variety of members, taking steps to reach consensus, introducing new topics, and ensuring that the team does not go too far over time limits for each agenda item.
- *Pull the group together if the discussion fragments into multiple conversations.* A team is not functioning as a whole when three groups are talking at once. The leader must stop such confusion quickly and, without being dictatorial, have one member speak at a time.

■ *Encourage input from all members.* All members have important ideas to impart; sometimes those who are the most quiet have the most interesting ideas. Perhaps they remain silent simply because their ideas seem different from everyone else's ideas. In any case, a leader can use several methods to draw out quiet members. One method is to go around the table, asking for brief comments from everyone. Another approach is to ask the quiet members directly for their ideas (for some members, this may be too threatening) or to ask these members for their ideas outside the meeting. In any case, the leader must validate the member's contribution, or he or she—and other quiet members—will be more likely to contribute as the process moves on.

■ *Prevent domination by one group member.* To remedy this problem, the leader can ask for short contributions from everyone, or from specific members. The leader can also put an arbitrary time limit on comments (at the risk of seeming too domineering). Another idea is for the leader to ask all members to write short comments anonymously, distribute them randomly around the table, and read them aloud. Perhaps one of the most effective remedies is for the leader to speak privately with the member dominating the group, politely asking him or her to allow others equal time.

■ *Check for consensus or group decisions.* The leader cannot make decisions for the group. He or she must guide the group through the sometimes difficult process of reaching a consensus decision. This may or may not be reached by a unanimous vote. Team decision making tools discussed on page 105 can be very helpful. Indeed, unanimity is rare and not necessarily desirable. Reaching consensus requires getting all members' views, building respect for various views, objectively weighing the implications of each view, and recognizing that rarely will a decision please all members.

■ *Finally, a team leader must work with the person or group overseeing the team to report its progress.* Such reports require the ability to summarize information supported by accurate records. The leader also delegates details such as keeping records and scheduling meetings, and may also coordinate any added education for members (for example, in indicator monitoring).

Recorder

As the name denotes, this member keeps a written record of meetings. He or she also can set or document agendas, compile minutes, and secure needed documents for the team. This assignment may not seem like a prize, but it is vital to efficient functioning; therefore, it should be rotated among members without considering rank in the organization.

Quality Expert

This member has special expertise in quality assessment and improvement; a project staff person may fit this role. This person should be familiar with quality improvement tools and have excellent teaching skills. If additional expertise is needed, the team may use consultants or other outside experts in statistics, engineering, market research, and so on.

Team Member

Ultimately, responsibility for a team's success rests with the members. Each member participates in discussion, performs specific assignments (such as data collection), contributes his or her expertise and creativity, and may help implement actions. Members also carry out specific roles (such as recorder or facilitator) as necessary. Although a team leader may be the most visible presence, each member must know that without his or her unique contribution, the process can falter. Quality improvement, after all, includes mutual respect and cooperation, about effective communication and removal of barriers.

▣ Team Stages

Getting Acquainted and Started

Perhaps little will be done to improve the quality of care delivery at this stage, but what takes place early in the team's life can determine how well it will function in the future. In this early stage, members become familiar with each other. Team members from diverse backgrounds may have had little direct communication in the past or may not have communicated as equals. Perhaps different constituent representatives sitting around the table harbor preconceived notions about each other, which will be tested during the getting-acquainted stage. Later in the group's life, these notions will probably be disproved.

Members will want to see how the team leader functions. Will he or she be dominant or passive? Will he or she be open to ideas from all members? Will the environment be constructive, destructive, invigorating, or stifling? Will the leader encourage all members to speak, or will he or she allow certain members to dominate discussions? Will the leader keep the group on track when it wanders? Does the leader have a hidden agenda?

In this early stage, members will often speak gingerly, testing the waters, waiting to see whether they will comfortably be able to speak their minds. Response from the leader and from other members at this tender stage will often determine the quality of later participation.

At first, the team will be unsure of its duties and goals. Members may be hopeful that improvement is possible or they may be skeptical about the entire process. At this stage, members should be encouraged to introduce themselves, share ideas openly, and define and explore the task at hand. The team should know that it will not make great strides in the first several meetings; this is the time for clarifying goals and becoming comfortable as a team.

Getting Underway

A team must go through certain growing pains and developmental stages. Even when the most competent and secure person or group tackles a large project, some fear occurs. The project looks too big, too complex. The people feel they do not have the time or the skills. Members may not be sure how to proceed: the first step is often the hardest to choose. Prejudices, hidden agendas, and other conflicts among team members may surface. Team members may be contentious; conversely, they may be overly polite. Neither is necessarily productive.

At this stage, teams may find the path to their goal obscure, and any spirit of optimism may wane. As in any relationship, the key is not jumping ship. If members can work through the panic and pain, the relationship becomes stronger; the members gain mutual respect. This stage can also be productive in terms of the improvement task at hand. If members initially thought a process was simple and easy to improve, this stage may bring the realization of how complex most processes are, particularly in behavioral health.

The earlier stages of team building may not show progress toward improving the quality of care delivery, but they are necessary for team growth and success. To get through this stage with the team intact, the leader needs to allow enough freedom for members to air their concerns, but should not let the group deteriorate into diatribes, war stories, or sullen silence. The leader must be especially skilled in the techniques that help groups create ideas and reach consensus. Above all, the leader must show faith in the process and must reassure the team that beyond the pain lies productivity.

Team Building

Having survived some difficulty, the group should emerge with renewed confidence and new interpersonal skills. At this point, a more cohesive group begins to form as members realize that the sum of the group can produce a better result than any individual effort. Previously competitive relationships become more cooperative, and individual agendas are adjusted to meet the group's needs. Disagreements are open and honest, and members actively listen to each other. Understanding, compromise, trust, and openness are the norm.

As a result, creative ideas begin to emerge, and members see real hope for improvement. In short, team members respect and accept each other, and they feel good about what they are doing as a team. At this stage, the leader must channel the energy into productive problem analysis and solving.

Team Work

Here is where the real work is accomplished. The team is now comfortable about settling conflicts or disagreements; it has established and become comfortable with its criteria and rules, and has begun to demonstrate true problem-solving behavior. At this stage, the team is also becoming more knowledgeable about the issues at hand: the care delivery network; structure, process, and outcome; indicator monitoring; and so on.

The leadership role changes at this point. If a firm hand was sometimes necessary in the previous steps, team members may now require less guidance. If a team needed motivation or reassurance before, it may have grown beyond that need. In fact, the team may now require slowing at times.

One pitfall of this stage is regression. Any number of circumstances can move a team back to a previous stage: loss of a member, new members, an unsuccessful test, or a new directive from a steering committee or administration. The leader may need to remind the group that regression is an expected part of the process.

In addition, all members should know that the duration and intensity of these stages will vary. A team that is not progressing the way it wants should not be demoralized; rather, it should understand that no progression at this stage is normal, and it should look for the tools necessary to improve the team's efforts.

▣ A Team Improvement Cycle

Once underway, improvement work with teams follows an improvement cycle. The following steps are adapted from *The Team Handbook:*

Clarify Goals

- Discuss mission statement
- Create an improvement plan

Educate and Build the Team

- Start building the team
- Set ground rules and logistics
- Discuss quality issues
- Educate team members about quality improvement tools

Investigate the Process

- Describe the process or problem
- Localize problems
- Look for root causes
- Test and refine data collection procedures

Analyze Data and Seek Solutions

- Look for patterns in the data
- Explore schematic solutions
- Develop a strategy for further improvement

Take Appropriate Action

- Loop back for further investigation
- Design or redesign the product or process
- Standardize procedures
- Stabilize the process
- Monitor the results of all changes—evaluate and refine as needed
- Document progress

Establish Closure

- Evaluate the team's process
- Evaluate the project's results
- Organize files
- Update picture book format
- Make final presentation
- Recommend follow-up activities

▣ Ingredients for a Successful Team

This section includes tips for creating and maintaining a successful team:

- *Identify team goals.* Members will need to know what will be expected from the project.
- *Prepare a mission statement.* With a mission statement, the team will understand its purpose, limitations, expectations, authority, composition, and structure.
- *Determine resources.* This will help the team know what education, budget, expertise, and so forth are needed.
- *Select the team leader.* Through whatever process the organization chooses, a leader who is knowledgeable, interested, and skilled should be selected.
- *Assign the project advisor.* If the advisor is different from the leader, this person should be identified.
- *Select project teams.* If sub-teams are required, they should be small (five members plus the leader and advisor) and composed of parties involved with the task at hand.
- *Use agendas.* Agendas will help keep meetings on track.
- *Use effective discussion skills.* These should include asking for clarification, listening, summarizing, minimizing digression, managing time, and testing for consensus.
- *Set up a record-keeping system.* Agendas, minutes, and documents are ways to track a team's work.

■ *Set group rules.* Matters such as attendance, promptness, meeting place and time, the importance of full participation, and so on should be decided up front.

Next, certain behaviors by participants foster effective team functioning. The following list is taken from *Teamwork in Cooperative Extension Programs:*

■ Participants communicate openly and nondefensively; they listen attentively.

■ Participants respect and trust each other, have confidence in each other's abilities, and support one another.

■ Participants allow and encourage equal participation and sharing of ideas, including expression of dissenting views.

■ Participants confront conflicts and problems; they use disagreement and conflict productively.

■ Participants are skillful in decision making and problem solving.

The following are some additional attributes found in successful teams:

■ Develop an improvement plan. An improvement plan helps the team determine what advice, assistance, training, materials, and other resources it may need.

■ Reward beneficial team behaviors. Encourage all members to use the skills and practices that make discussions and meetings effective.

■ Participants believe in and are committed to the value of working together in a spirit of cooperation.

■ Team size is appropriate for effective communication.

■ Participants understand the overall objectives of the project.

■ Participants understand individual roles and responsibilities, as well as relationships to other staff members.

■ Participants take the time to establish and clarify guidelines and procedures for a working relationship; they are committed to making plans and achieving them.

- Participants define and agree on meaningful and measurable objectives that meet both group and personal needs; individuality and creativity are not stifled.

- Someone within the group assumes leadership to coordinate each task or program effort.

- Participants function well in a variety of roles (initiating, informing, summarizing, mediating, encouraging) and know when appropriate roles are needed.

- Participants know each other. That is, they are aware of each other's resources, skills, and expertise. They know what each person can contribute to the group.

- The group allows sufficient time for the teamwork effort.

- The group places work first, but also allows social interaction.

▣ References

Scholtes PR: *The Team Handbook: How to Use Teams to Improve Quality*. Madison, WI: Joiner Associates, Inc, 1988.

Teamwork in Cooperative Extension Programs. Madison, WI: University of Wisconsin, 1980.

Using Quality Improvement Tools in a Health Care Setting. Oakbrook Terrace, IL: Joint Commission, 1992.

Appendix

C

101 Quality Principles

1. Let the data tell the story; data "pictures" are vital.

2. Provide larger time blocks to project teams; two to four hours at a minimum; consider all-day workshops.

3. Use a guide for structured meetings; do not deviate! Use role assignments consistently (for example, appoint a time keeper and a facilitator).

4. Whenever possible, use staff leadership for quality project teams.

5. Select team members whose skills and background are appropriate for the problems they are to address.

6. Keep graphic displays of the problem-solving process and quality improvement process posted everywhere.

7. Always have a full set of quality tools available for project teams (for example, flip chart).

8. Keep detailed minutes of quality project teams, but use an action-oriented format. Don't forget key assignments and the person responsible.

9. Keep working; don't give up.

10. Provide time for quality activities; you cannot do this in "extra" or "leftover" time.

11. Teach staff the scientific method (concept, hypothesis, data collection, analysis, and evaluation).

12. Use a "just in time" method to train as many staff as possible, as quickly as possible, in quality methods.

13. Develop a quality mentor system to help further support emerging teams and quality philosophy.

14. Praise, praise, praise real accomplishments.

15. Reinforce and identify elements of the new culture (for example, manager as teacher).

16. Link all quality activities to real demands and real problems in the environment.

17. Do not accept redundancy.

18. Demand excellence, but not perfection.

19. Allow staff to try, and expect failure—but expect staff to continue trying.

20. Join critical functions in quality cluster projects (for example, staff development with ongoing quality projects on budget planning).

21. Project teams should always mix staff from all levels of the organization, including support, management, and administration.

22. Stay on time lines—quality activities must be a priority—you must perform what you set out to do.

23. Establish a quality resource center for data collection, especially for survey design and analysis.

24. Reinforce long-term commitment with short and intermediate success.

25. Keep the sponsors of quality projects informed, involved, and focused on the process and outcome of quality project teams.

26. Develop a strategic plan for implementation of quality projects over the next year; too many projects will overwhelm the organization and too few will not establish the cultural change.

27. Post quality activities in prominent locations (for example, project team story boards near the cafeteria).

28. Establish an annual quality fair or celebration.

29. Adopt a model of continuous performance feedback—annual performance evaluations are inadequate.

30. Reinforce staff for doing the right thing correctly.

31. Institute required reading on the quality philosophy.

32. Live, breathe, and embrace the concept of customer satisfaction.

33. You must value your employees and yourself to produce the right work environment to achieve total customer satisfaction.

34. Give each employee maximum degrees of freedom and autonomy to produce the highest quality output.

35. Develop a compensation program for employees that brings together monetary rewards, a flexible work environment, organization ownership, and leadership opportunities.

36. Develop and foster a corporate identity that is synonymous with quality.

37. Give employees maximum freedom to "fix" problems at the local level.

38. Break down organization-based hierarchies and barriers, and reconfigure your staff structure around work processes.

39. Define (in detail!) all work processes.

40. Study (in detail!) all work processes.

41. Know thyself! Know thy customer!

42. Accept no excuses—expect errors to occur and continually correct them.

43. Look for your absolute worst areas of performance; start with your most significant problems and dissect them with cause-and-effect diagrams.

44. Keep a performance track record of quality project group involvements and continually show them to staff and customers.

45. Establish a customer-centered database and update it continuously.

46. Benchmark! Benchmark! Benchmark! Study the best work processes where you find them and continually adopt them.

47. A work process is what you do—it is the vital function of your organization.

48. Develop an overall quality index based on all your project team outcomes and continuous quality improvement paybacks.

49. Use all available analysis tools, particularly those that combine results, such as meta-analysis, to help in benchmarking (for example, pooled analysis of existing data).

50. Reinforce (consistently) top management involvement, commitment and long-term vision of quality culture.

51. Enlist quality disbelievers in quality activities that have a direct bearing on the quality of their work life.

52. Form local and national networks of quality organizations to share data and support cross-organization change.

53. Examine your organization's suppliers and require their participation in quality activities or change your suppliers.

54. Examine your outside referrals and require their participation in quality activities.

55. Require each service area to define its customers (internal, external) and identify (in detail!) all relevant customer requirements.

56. Build customer requirements into the goals and objectives of the organization.

57. Keep the customer!

58. Treat every job in the work environment as equally important.

59. Treat every employee in the work environment as equally important.

60. Use all of the quality rituals at your disposal.

61. Pick a quality improvement process that fits the problem (for example, total quality management project teams versus performance management initiatives versus continuous quality improvement actions).

62. Invest in cause-and-effect thinking! This essentially establishes one of the fundamentals for the problem-solving process and provides a detailed dissection of work processes.

63. Give up the "end stage" inspection model as a method to improve quality; this approach may still have limited application for gross error-rate detection.

64. Believe and act in concert with the belief that continuous quality improvement is essential for the survival of the organization.

65. Accept that people close to the work processes have the best data and ideas as to how to improve them.

66. Accept and believe that most people in your organization are eager to work competently and will perform at the highest level if given the opportunity.

67. Invest in consultants (internal or external) to develop reliable and valid data collection approaches, including design of surveys and subsequent analysis.

68. Give staff adequate training in both the logistics and methods of quality, but also in the philosophy of quality.

69. Do not fight the quality "jargon"—it is part of and signals the ongoing organizational change.

70. Indoctrinate new employees in the quality method from the beginning. Make it part of the orientation to your organization and first week's employee basic training.

71. Make it mandatory that all staff participate in quality project teams or continuous quality improvement initiatives.

72. Be ready to help managers and administrators begin the process of change to new roles, including teaching.

73. Study and use the specialized quality techniques.

74. Follow quality, and the dollars will come to you; chase the dollars, and you will compromise the quality.

75. Build loyalty through commitment to your basic values and continually demonstrate your commitment to quality.

76. Listen to your customers—surveys, complaints, conversations, and referral sources can give you a world of information.

77. Tolerate skepticism, but not disrespect, of quality theories.

78. Build a cost/benefit, benefit/cost model of quality initiatives and track your organization success.

79. Require presentations by staff of quality initiatives to your top administrative and governance structures.

80. Read sociological books and collections of unobtrusive measures (for example, study natural pedestrian crosswalks prior to putting in sidewalks!).

81. Ask questions and listen, listen, listen.

82. Leaders must be teachers, designers, and mentors.

83. End the practice of "inspection" as a quality control measure.

84. Change the way departments treat each other—make client flow seamless.

85. Expect resistance to change.

86. Make good work processes better.

87. Continuously measure outcomes data.

88. Use "quality by design" thinking.

89. Realize the complexity of outcomes measures—they integrate client experience.

90. Recognize that quality comes in many forms.

91. Adopt, articulate, and measure a philosophy of care.

92. Select a small number of critical work processes to improve—at first.

93. Form a limited number of well-trained, field ready project teams—at first.

94. Consistently work to close performance gaps.

95. Collect useful data—not all data everywhere!

96. Listen to your data; understand your data.

97. Use cross functional, cross departmental, cross discipline teams, and indicators.

98. Provide adequate time for training and quality improvement work.

99. Bring enthusiasm!

100. Don't stop!

101. Be open and honest!

Index